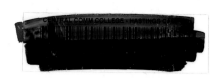

RIGHT TO RECOVER

Winning the Political and Religious Wars over Stem Cell Research in America

Yvonne Perry

©2007
Nightengale Press
A Nightengale Media LLC Company

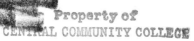
RIGHT TO RECOVER

The information in this book is not meant to be construed as any type of medical advice or as making promises that a cure will definitely be found using stem cells of any kind. This is a compilation of research material and the author's opinion about stem cell research only. Those quoted in this book have given their full permission to be quoted, and all references used in compiling the information found in this book are listed in the Bibliography.

For information about Nightengale Press please
visit our website at www.nightengalepress.com.
Email: publisher@nightengalepress.biz
or send a letter to:
Nightengale Press
10936 N. Port Washington Road. Suite 206
Mequon, WI 53092
Library of Congress Cataloging-in-Publication Data

Perry, Yvonne,
    RIGHT TO RECOVER/ Yvonne Perry
ISBN:1-933449-41-1
ISBN:978-1-933449-41-8
Non-Fiction

Copyright Registered: 2007
First Published by Nightengale Press in the USA

October 2007
10 9 8 7 6 5 4 3 2 1
Printed in the United States of America

Endorsements

"Yvonne Perry's book enrages and inspires: it leaves you with the feeling that something must be done, that it can be done, and that it will be done—because we will do it. This book changes the equation."

—Don C. Reed, Roman Reed Spinal Cord Injury Research Act

It is such a pleasure to work with a writer like Yvonne Perry. She has truly researched the research and spent hundreds of hours to find the facts to share with the readers of *RIGHT TO RECOVER.*

Over the years I have read literally thousands of articles and documents from around the world about this subject and *RIGHT TO RECOVER* is the most complete work I have ever read. It provides an honest evaluation and asks readers to consider the facts and then form their own opinion instead of listening to people who have never researched the subject.

—Reverend Dan Bloodworth,
The Brian Bloodworth Stroke and Head Injury Research Foundation

In a world confused with chaos in regard to stem cell research, Yvonne Perry has moved beyond the political to the healing in her new book *RIGHT TO RECOVER Winning the Political and Religious Wars over Stem Cell Research in America.* This educational book sheds light on the way Americans view embryonic stem cell research and provides well-researched facts about all types of stem cell treatments throughout the world. This book will shed light on the future, today.

—*Dr. Eric S. Kaplan, Author of Dying to be Young, From Botox to Botulism and Lifestyles of the Fit and Famous*

Finally, the truth about stem cell research. I search the Internet daily for articles on stem cell research to pass along to other advocates. It's so maddening to constantly read the opposition's blatant lies concerning stem cell research.

—*Diane Wyshak, Stem Cell Battles.com*

When I started reading *RIGHT TO RECOVER Winning the Political and Religious Wars over Stem Cell Research in America,* I thought it would be interesting and that as an Executive Director of a healthcare not-for-profit dealing with this issue, I might glean some new knowledge. The book delivered far more than I ever expected. I was completely hooked by it from beginning to end. The author, Yvonne Perry, does an excellent job in defining stem cell research and in making the case for funding of the different types of stem cell research, especially blastocyst (or embryonic) stem cell research. I highly recommend *RIGHT TO RECOVER* to those who are sitting on the fence with this issue.

—*Cherie Fisher for Reader Views*

Yvonne Perry counters long-standing myths of the American stem cell debate with bright, accessible prose. Policymakers and everyday citizens who want to make informed choices about stem cell research need to read *RIGHT TO RECOVER.*

—*Shane G. Smith, Ph.D., Science Director, CNS Foundation, Former Science Director, 'Yes on Proposition 71'*

Dedication

This book is dedicated to all those who suffer with an illness or injury that might be cured or alleviated through stem cell technology; to all the doctors and scientists who do the biological research; to all those who have privately funded or lobbied for a more flexible policy on blastocyst stem cell research.

Acknowledgements

Chuck McCann – thank you for sharing your story. You are an inspiration to those who take life for granted.

Don C. Reed (California's Proposition 71) – thank you for checking my facts, editing my text and allowing me to quote you. You spent an entire weekend reading this manuscript to make sure my thoughts and research are presented in the best light possible. Thank you for connecting me with Dr. Shane Smith, Rayilyn Brown, Frank Cocazzelli, Nina Brown, and so many more people who made this book the factual work it is. Your help brought this book to a superb level of credibility.

Doris Mauldin – More than a mother, more than a friend, you are my best fan and quite the proofreader!

Dr. Aaron Milstone – thank you for believing in me yet again and for helping me contact key people at Vanderbilt University Medical Center.

Dr. Evan Snyder – thank you for writing the foreword of the book and for enduring my numerous phone calls and emails. Thank you for all the research you do to help others live a healthier life.

Dr. James Fallon – thank you for bearing with me while I asked many questions.

Dr. Madan Jagasia – thank you for a most informative interview on this fascinating subject. Thank you for all your help.

Dr. Shane Smith, Ph.D. Science Director of the Children's

Neurobiological Solutions Foundation (advocate for California's Proposition 71) – thank you for taking time out of your busy schedule to review my facts and help me edit this work. Your hours of patient reading and red-lining are so much appreciated.

Frank Cocazzelli (Institute for Progressive Christianity) – You showed me a side of religion I was unaware of. What an eye-opener. Thank you for checking my facts and guiding me to be more tolerant.

Heather Scott – Thank you for contacting Alicia Mattson, Chair of Libertarian Party of Tennessee to gain her position statement. Thank you, Alicia.

Joan Stewart, the Publicity Hound – thank you for helping me spread the word about my stem cell survey.

Linda Wyshak – thank you for all your endless searching to find information I needed. Your work to help others is much appreciated.

Maggie Goldberg – thank you for sharing the Christopher Reeve Foundation's position statement.

Mary Schneider – thank you for sharing your story and for all you do to help others understand the value of blastocyst stem cell research. Thank you for connecting me with Dr. Kurtzberg.

Michael Davis – this is for you and all those who suffer. May you be well.

Nina Brown – thank you for sharing your story and excellent information with me.

Randy Perry – thank you for bearing with me during the long hours of writing this book. You have endured endless hours of "alone" time while I was typing away in my office.

Rayilyn Brown – What would I have done without you and all your help? You are such a trooper. In spite of your own suffering, you are always thinking of others and fighting for recovery. Thank you for connecting me with all the other wonderful people on the PD listserv.

Reverend Dan Bloodworth – thank you for your years of stem cell research and for standing in faith to help others understand blastocyst stem cell research.

Shonna Hyde – thank you for connecting me with Dr. Snyder

and giving him countless messages on my behalf.

Stephanie Bowen - for connecting me with Maggie Goldberg.

Susan Fajt — thank you for sharing your story. Your loss is great, but your spirit is greater. I am inspired by your willingness to help others recover.

Taryn Simpson - for sharing your story, your friendship and for being the blessing you are to me.

Valerie Connelly at Nightengale Press - my publisher is now also my dear friend!

CONTENT

DEDICATION

ACKNOWLEDGEMENTS

FOREWORD by Dr. Evan Snyder

INTRODUCTION

1. Basic Overview of Stem Cell Research   18
2. Why All the Controversy?   36
3. Biblical Support for Blastocystic Research   59
4. Separation of Church and State   70
5. Rebuttal of President Bush's Statement   94
6. What Does Cloning Have to Do with Stem Cell Research?   111
7. National Research   120
8. International Research   150
9. Public Opinion about Stem Cell Research   172
10. The Significance of Federal Funding   198
11. Challenging the Prentice List   216
12. Possible Cures from Stem Cell Research   250
13. Turning the Tides Toward the *RIGHT TO RECOVER*   282

APPENDIX   296

BIBLIOGRAPHY A   306

BIBLIOGRAPHY B   321

ABOUT THE AUTHOR   334

Foreword by Dr. Evan Snyder

I first learned of Yvonne Perry and her work when she approached me at the suggestion of Reverend Dan Bloodworth. He and I had been in touch many times during his quest for more information about stem cell research that might help his son regain use of his body. I knew there would probably come a day when Dan would do something with all the information he had gathered, so it didn't surprise me that he would pair with a writer who shares our passion for the research. I was surprised when Yvonne traveled from Nashville, Tennessee to La Jolla, California to visit me here at Burnham Institute for Medical Research and asked me to write the foreword for her book. I am pleased to be part of this effort to help people better understand all types of stem cell research.

Throughout the writing of *RIGHT TO RECOVER, Winning the Political and Religious Wars over Stem Cell Research in America*, Yvonne consulted with me and many other scientists and knowledgeable people to make sure she got her facts straight. I appreciate her tenacity to deliver accurate biological information. Upon reading the galley copy, I am equally impressed with her personal logic and historical account of how politics and religion have been superimposed upon the landscape of scientific research. Yvonne has already received a fair share of criticism for her stand on research on stem cells derived from blastocysts; all the more reason her book is so valuable at this point. People have been exposed to too much misinformation, and the research has endured enough setbacks in legislation due to unfounded beliefs that simply play into political agendas. I have found that when provided with correct data, the public responds in a logical manner, typically, supportive of this area of investigation.

The book you are holding speaks to the stem cell research issue, going beyond the scientific scene and putting the research into a societal context. It's written for the layperson, who may not follow the field in detail, but wants to find out what's happening beneath the surface. This book will teach you the facts and hit on issues the average citizen would like to know in order to make informed decisions regarding stem cell research—especially with so many states offering the opportunity to vote on legislation that affects its use. Yvonne has thoroughly covered each aspect from every angle and made a good case for why all types of stem cell research should be federally funded.

You can use this book as a resource for understanding the biology as well as the religious and political "who, what, and why", surrounding all types of stem cell research. For example, if you want to know more about an individual or topic, you have heard on a talk show, you will more than likely find that information in this book. Do you want to know whether adult or pre-implantation stem cells are more effective? Do you need a tutorial on definitions? All this is readily found in this book.

The word "embryonic" when referring to stem cell research is unfortunate. It conjures one meaning for scientists and another thing for the lay public. The word is so imprecise that the lay public automatically thinks of "babies". Obviously, this is very far from reality. A discussion of embryology, as Yvonne attempts, makes this clear.

Scientists and researchers are finding more uses for blastocyst stem cells than solely cell replacement (although, this is the use most prominently discussed in the media). These amazing cells can be used to reduce scarring and inflammation; they offer factors that can protect cells and stimulate growth, and can even be used to detoxify our bodies by soaking up poisons.

The science is quite young and changes from month to month. In fact, the field of stem cell research changes so rapidly that no matter how up-to-date you want to be. By the time a sentence appears on a printed page, it may be outdated. The theories we accept as truth today, will be thought ridiculous and obsolete tomorrow. However, this field of research is doing exactly what science should be doing. It's like intellectual ping-pong match among researchers. One person throws out an idea, it carries for a little bit over the net, and then someone looks at it and bats it back and says, "No, you're wrong." Then, another person counters with data that supports another argument. Which side of the net the ping-pong ball is on changes from week to week? We don't know because it is constantly changing and going back and forth. One group will say you can get stem cells from the pancreas; another group will say, "No, you did the research wrong." Then, another group will say, "No, you did your counter-proof incorrectly." Each adds information without necessarily establishing a winner or loser.

We can't say that anything has been established as an absolute and irrefutable truth about stem cells, but it is safe to say that, in the body, there are cells that are very plastic. Beyond that, I'm not sure there is anything in the stem cell field that we can say has been proven with 100 percent certainty. Even so, Yvonne Perry has made a tremendous effort to offer the most up-to-date and factual information on stem cell research as possible at this time. Her presentation can be trusted to bring people to a better understanding of the field of stem cell research and the issues surrounding it.

For the lay public, this book is more accessible, comprehensive and filled with more than any other book on stem cell research presently on the market. It is with satisfaction and great honor that I endorse *RIGHT TO RECOVER*.

Introduction

I met Reverend Dan Bloodworth in 2005 and immediately became intrigued by his enthusiasm regarding stem cell research. Dan's All-American athlete son, Brian, suffered a spinal cord injury when he was hit by lightning in 1987. Motivated by his desire to find a treatment that would allow his son to communicate and become mobile again, Dan has devoted 16 years of his life to learn everything he could about stem cell research and share that information with anyone willing to listen. I am inspired by this ordinary man who believes he can make the world a better place by helping others understand the facts about this controversial issue.

While working with Michael Davis on his book, *FROM TRAGEDY TO TRIUMPH: A Personal Story about Living with Quadriplegia,* I became keenly aware of, and very interested in, the healing potential that blastocyst (also known as embryonic) stem cell research offers victims of spinal cord injury, Parkinson's disease, Alzheimer's, cancer, renal failure, paralysis, heart disease, and many other illnesses. By diligently using his communication skills to secure equal rights for persons with disabilities, Mr. Davis, battling quadriplegia himself, has made an impact on the way disadvantaged citizens are treated. Michael Davis is determined to help as many people as possible in any way he can. I am inspired by this man confined to a wheelchair who has impacted society in such a positive manner.

While I was assisting Michael with his book, H.R. 810 (the

Stem Cell Research Enhancement Act of 2005) was passed by Congress. Supporters held their breath while they hoped and prayed that funds would be released for blastocyst stem cell research. Influenced by the opinion of narrow-minded politicians and members of the religious community, President Bush's decision to veto H.R. 810 had a heartbreaking impact on members of our society who have physical and medical disabilities. His decision and the mindset of the misinformed right-wing ultra-orthodox party must be challenged if our society is to benefit from blastocyst stem cell biotechnology. And that is why I wrote this book.

RIGHT TO RECOVER is an educational book created in hopes of shedding light upon, and making a difference in, the way we view blastocyst stem cell biology. I am not a doctor or scientist specializing in a particular field of research; I am a planetary healer and global citizen involved in bringing peace and goodwill to humankind. I have been blessed with a talent for writing, communication, and technical research, which I use daily to enlighten and strengthen my fellow sojourners. You will need to keep an open mind while reading and pondering this book. Otherwise, your ego may become offended before your spirit has a chance to process the information.

RIGHT TO RECOVER contains well-researched facts about all types of stem cell technology and lends insight into the political and religious issues surrounding blastocyst stem cell technology. The book covers bone marrow, amniotic and cord blood stem cell treatments presently being used and their restorative effects. It also explores the use of blastocyst stem cell technology on laboratory animals, and presents findings to support the curative potential of this technology on humans. I've used Biblical references to show why a 12- to 48-hour-old mass of human cells is NOT a human being and how God has given us stem cell technology as a scientific gift for healing. As you can tell from the bibliography, the information in this book was derived from intensive research, personal interviews, emails, and other correspondence with national and international medical doctors, research scientists, religious leaders, and elected officials. I have included stories from patients who hope to transform their lives through cures or treatments derived from stem cell research.

The topic of stem cell research is making headlines in every country. You may have read articles and heard stories that are not exactly true. *RIGHT TO RECOVER* will not present you with glossed over fairy tales about how stem cells can miraculously cure any disease, and it will not promote fear-based rumors you may have heard from the pulpit on Sunday. This book is factual and is the result of at least 400 hours of Internet searching, article reading, face-to-face interviews, emails, and phone calls with scientific experts on all types of stem cell research.

The landscape in this field changes very quickly as new breakthroughs are reported almost daily. Therefore, some of the material in this book may be outdated by the time it is published. I recommend that you visit www.right2recover.com periodically to check for new material.

Stem cell technology should not be the political or religious issue it has become. Every decision maker should investigate scientifically proven facts before making a decision regarding any issue that affects other people. Those who oppose stem cell research do not have all the facts. It is my hope to inform readers and bring about an understanding that will remove the stumbling blocks and release funds for all types of stem cell and biotech research in the US. We all have the *RIGHT TO RECOVER*.

RIGHT
TO
RECOVER

Chapter One

BASIC OVERVIEW OF STEM CELL RESEARCH

Stem cell research is being actively conducted around the world for both scientific and medical reasons. Scientifically, stem cell biology provides excellent information about what is normal and abnormal regarding how cells develop. Understanding what causes cells to become diseased helps scientists find ways to prevent genes from becoming dysfunctional. It also helps them produce drugs and treatments to cure illnesses. Medically, adult stem cells from bone marrow and human umbilical cord blood have been proven to repair and regenerate diseased cells when transplanted into animals and humans. Never in history has one technology held such strong potential to help a majority of people live a healthier life as does the science of stem cell biology. Likewise, never in history has such a remarkable science been so ethically debated.

There are two categories of stem cells: adult and embryonic. For clarification in this book, the term "adult stem cells" refers to stem cells harvested from umbilical cord blood, the placenta, amniotic fluid drawn during pregnancy, and bone marrow of a child or fully-grown adult. The term "embryonic stem cells" refers to stem cells harvested from fertilized eggs created *in vitro* (outside the body).

What is a Stem Cell?

Stem cells are an undifferentiated group of cells which, depending on their surrounding conditions, are capable of developing into other types of cells such as liver cells, kidney cells, brain cells, or any of the other 260 different types of cells that make up the human body.

There are three types of stem cells: totipotent, which can develop into an entire embryo; pluripotent, which undergo a process of differentiation that changes them into multipotent cells (also called unipotent); and multipotent, which give rise to cells that have a particular function. Multipotent cells (adult stem cells) are permanently differentiated or fixed. For example, multipotent blood stem cells give rise to red blood cells, white blood cells, and platelets, but they cannot functionally develop into other non-blood cells such as liver cells, nerve cells, or heart muscle cells. These unique cells are with us throughout our lives and are used by the body to repair unhealthy or disabled cells of like kind.

Stem cells respond to the other cells around them, and a cell's fate is determined by the other cells and chemicals in its environment. In their natural state, both totipotent and pluripotent stem cells are not yet any type of cell; instead, they are unassigned or blank. These "undifferentiated" cells have no specific purpose assigned to them other than to reproduce like cells while waiting for a genetic signal to tell them to develop into another type of cell. These signals are found within the environment of the body. Biologists are learning about these signals in hopes of determining the molecular method these stem cells use to differentiate and become tissues, nerves, vessels, and organs. It is believed that organs and tissues may one day be grown from pluripotent cells in laboratories to be used in lieu of, or in addition to, human organ donation. However, the main reason scientists study totipotent and pluripotent cells is to learn more about the cells' behavior. Understanding what causes cells to become diseased will help researchers know how to produce drugs and treatments to combat or even prevent disease.

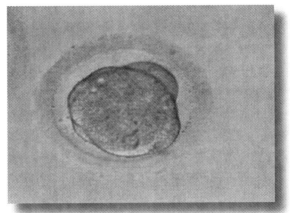

Morula Photo Courtesy of Dr. Ric Ross

When a sperm and ovum are united (whether *in vitro* or inside the female body) fertilization occurs, and the two parts become a single totipotent cell. A fertilized egg is also known as a zygote. Within hours after fertilization this cell divides into two identical cells, which also divide thus forming pluripotent stem cells. By the fourth day the cell cluster has divided to reach approximately 16 cells, and it is called a morula. The division/multiplication process continues for about five days until a hollow sphere of about 32 cells is formed along with a fluid-filled cavity. This sphere or cluster of primordial cells is then called a blastocyst.

RIGHT TO RECOVER—*Yvonne Perry*

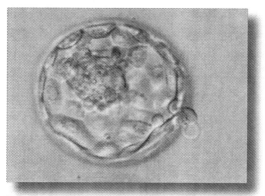

Blastocyst Photo Courtesy of Dr. Ric Ross

If the blastocyst cells are inside the womb, development continues as these stem cells begin to differentiate and form all the cells needed to make an entire human being. However, in an artificial environment outside the body (in vitro), the pluripotent stem cells from a fertilized egg will only reproduce more undifferentiated cells. They cannot produce a fully developed embryo.

A blastocyst has an inner and outer layer of cells. The outer layer (called the trophectoderm) will form the placenta and other tissue needed to support development in the uterus. The inner cells are undifferentiated or unspecific in what they will become, but they are able to form any type of cell found in a human body. If the entire blastocyst is inserted into the uterus, it must implant itself and begin to draw nourishment from the mother in order to move to the next stage of development. If implantation (conception) occurs, the resulting embryo will become a fetus at eight weeks, which will develop into a human baby within nine months.

Within the womb a blastocyst automatically stops producing undifferentiated stem cells once the body parts have formed. Otherwise, a human would have multiple heads, hearts, legs, etc.

However, the inner cells of the blastocyst, if separated from the trophectoderm outside the uterus, cannot form an entire organism. These inner cells can continue to make more undifferentiated stem cells if properly tended to in a lab. The blastocysts used for stem cell research are cultured in lab containers outside the human body where a single cell may continue to divide up to 100 times. These newly developed undifferentiated cells are what researchers are studying.

Scientists do not know how long a cultured line of stem cells can continue to divide or live outside the uterus. The newly divided cells are used to study what causes undifferentiated stem cells to develop into particular cells. There is great hope of being able to cause these undifferentiated stem cells to form tissue, nerve cells, and organs that can be used for patients needing heart, lung, liver, and kidney transplants. Unlike human organ donors, who must die before their parts can be used by another human, the inner cells of the blastocyst may continue to create new living cells that might be used to make new organs, nerves, and tissues. By taking only one cell from the inner mass of the blastocyst, a new cell can be created. The remaining cells are not harmed. The blastocyst with one cell removed could theoretically be implanted into a uterus and brought to full term.

Stem Cell Technology Currently in Use

In my hope to have you accept all types of stem cell research, I'd like to show some ways that stem cell research is already benefiting society. At the top of the list are bone marrow transplants and umbilical cord blood infusions.

Bone Marrow Transplants

While its use is still in the developing stages, there are technologies available using adult stem cells to help people with heart conditions, spinal cord injuries, and orthopedic repair of bone and cartilage. Known as regenerative medicine, these techniques harness the body's natural ability to renew and heal itself. Here are a few examples:

- Here in the state of Tennessee, doctors at Vanderbilt University Medical Center commonly use bone marrow transplants in the treatment of cancer patients. More about that in just a moment.

- In Germany, heart attack victims have made a rapid and remarkable recovery after receiving implants of their own bone marrow stem cells during heart surgery.

- Mesoblast Limited is an Australian biotechnology company known for developing treatments through adult stem cell technology aimed at the regeneration and repair of bone and cartilage. In a pilot clinical trial at the Royal Melbourne Hospital, Mesoblast's technology was used on a patient with a 5cm fracture of the femur that had failed to heal after nine months. Three months after specialized stem cell treatment, the gap had been filled with new bone and the patient had regained use of his leg and was walking unaided.

Vanderbilt University Medical Center in Nashville specializes in adult stem cell transplant using either a patient's own stem cells, the stem cells of a related or unrelated donor, or cord blood stem cells to assist patients. The donor in sixty percent of all cases is a brother, sister, or adequately matched donor; however, there are cases where stem cells from an unrelated donor are used.

There are "cell banks" in the U.S. where hospitals may conduct a computerized search to locate the appropriate units and have them transported to the hospital where a patient is to receive treatment.

The blood-forming (hematopoietic) stem cells of bone marrow change into red, white, and other blood cells throughout life. The standard procedure for cancer treatment takes stem cells from the bone marrow of a patient. One way to retrieve them is to sedate the donor and stick needles in the hip bone and draw out the bone marrow. This method removes plasma, blood, and other cells, but a small population will be stem cells.

Because stem cells in the bone marrow are very small in quantity, recent technology gives the donor an injection prior to harvesting, to increase stem cell production so that it fills the marrow and spills into the blood. The blood is then drawn from a vein in one arm and pumped into a filter very much like a dialysis machine where the stem cells are spun at a certain speed causing the blood cells to separate into their components. Plasma will rise to the top, red cells will stick to the bottom, and the frothy looking layer in between is where the white cells and stem cells are trapped. The machine siphons off the stem cells and collects them before returning the rest of the blood to the vein in the donor's other arm. The entire closed-circuit cycle takes four to five hours and does no harm to the patient. Once the stem cells are obtained, they are frozen at 220 degrees below zero Fahrenheit until time to reintroduce them to the patient once chemotherapy is complete.

Each cancer disorder has its own stem cell. Some are so resilient they survive certain types of chemotherapy. There may be a pseudo cure or remission between times, but within a few years these cells may grow back and give rise to cancer again. In order to completely destroy the cancer stem cells the patient needs super high doses of chemotherapy. This concentrated dosage not only destroys cancer cells, it also destroys vital bone marrow cells in the process. It also destroys brain cells according to Dr. Mark Noble, Ph.D., an advocate in the field of stem cell research at University of Rochester Medical Center. Since this would result in death, high dosages cannot be used unless the patient's bone marrow cells are replaced afterward. Once chemotherapy is complete, the patient's own stem cells are reintroduced into the body where they regenerate perfectly healthy bone marrow cells and long-term health is restored to the patient. In my interview with Dr. Madan Jagasia, Assistant Professor of Medicine at Vanderbilt University Medical Center, he remarked, "We are basically rescuing patients using their own stem cells."

Another case where stem cells might be used is to restore a patient's heart muscle. When a patient has a heart attack, heart muscle is lost. You can balloon or stint the arteries, or do a by-pass operation, but once the heart muscle is lost it does not have the capacity to regenerate. Studies in Europe have been done where the patient's own stem cells are collected within two or three days after a heart attack and then purified and injected directly into the heart through catheters. The data from early animal and human studies show that these stem cells in the environment of the heart should be able to turn into heart muscle cells to repair or replace damaged cells.

Vanderbilt University Medical Center was the first hospital in the state of Tennessee to perform a new therapy using bone marrow stem cells to stimulate regeneration of the heart muscle after a heart attack. Douglas Vaughan, M.D., chief of the Division of Cardiovascular Medicine, reported that John Plummer, 63, underwent the stem cell regeneration therapy on March 11, 2007, after experiencing a heart attack one week prior. More randomized-controlled trials to study the effects of cell therapy in treating cardiac disease are scheduled.

Cord Blood

An Illinois mother Mary Schneider banked her son's cord blood when he was born. Within a year or so Ryan was showing moderate signs of cerebral palsy. By age two, the child only weighed 25 pounds and was unable to eat. His upper body strength was severely decreased, and he had only a two-word vocabulary. After nine months of speech therapy, his vocabulary consisted of 40 words, but he still had no sentence structure. Only close family members could understand him. Mary worried that her son's condition would only get worse. Hoping that regenerative stem cells would help him, Mary began the search for a doctor or biologist who could administer her son's cord blood CD34 stem cells back to him. Since the blood contained Ryan's own unaltered DNA and no drugs, the infusion process does not require FDA approval. It is an intravenous procedure. It should be simple, right?

Wrong. The search proved more difficult than Mary expected because the treatment using cord blood was so new it hadn't been tested, and many doctors were unwilling to take the risk without the support of clinical trials. After weeks of searching the Internet and making phone calls to leading stem cell researchers nationwide, Mary found little hope or information but a lot of refusals to do the transfusion. In an age when a patient can get donated blood from a stranger during surgery, no one would give this child his own cord blood! One doctor told Mary that he could give him Botox injections if Ryan's hands got too spastic!

Mary talked with Dr. Evan Snyder who deals mostly with

research using fetal and *in vitro* blastocyst stem cells. At the time (2005) Snyder's research was about five years away from human clinical trials. Mary couldn't wait that long. Upon Dr. Snyder's advice, she arranged for a metabolic study, a chromosome work up to conclude that Ryan did indeed have mild cerebral palsy and to establish a base-line study for comparison after the infusion. Pre- and post-infusion evaluations and progress monitoring with neural behavior experts and therapists were conducted through Easter Seals Dupage County, Illinois.

Dr. Harris, head of the Cord Blood Registry bank where Ryan's stem cells were stored, suggested Mary contact Dr. Joanne Kurtzberg, a pediatric oncologist in the Blood and Marrow Transplantation Division at Duke University, to see if she would do the infusion. Dr. Kurtzberg was willing to give the procedure a try, but she knew that, regardless of whether the treatment was successful or not, it would open the doors to a whole new dimension of the medical world, and she would be bombarded by the media and other researchers. In October 2005, just weeks prior to his third birthday, Dr. Kurtzberg introduced stem cells from Ryan's own cord blood to his body through a 20-minute intravenous drip of stem cells in the back of his hand. This was followed by two hours of saline drip to nudge the cells through his system. The cells then instinctively knew how to find their place and begin repair and regeneration. Within a week Ryan was showing progress and continued to improve in the weeks and months afterward. Eight months after the infusion, the dexterity in Ryan's hands and arms returned. Today the 4-year-old boy speaks clearly in coherent sentences and is at normal weight for his age group. He is testing at normal or even above average levels in motor skill tests.

Since there are so few studies on cord blood infusion, it can't be considered a proven treatment; therefore, insurance companies typically refuse to pay for the procedure. Mary Schneider went all the way to Capitol Hill to make sure other parents could access the treatment for their own children. She volunteers her time to train parents about what to expect during the procedure and the following months. She lobbied for federal funding for all types of stem cell research, hoping to receive grant money for parents who cannot afford the infusion their children need. Making speeches with Senator Brownback, Mary was in the East Room when President Bush vetoed H.R. 810. Five minutes before his announcement she had urged him not to veto the bill that would have expanded funding for blastocystic stem cell research. Then she sat in silent protest as the president vetoed the bill.

If you want to bank your child's cord blood, you have a choice of private or public banking options. Private banks will insure (for a fee) that your child's cord blood will be available whenever it is called for. Public banks do not charge for cord blood, but it is considered a donation to society and may be used by others who need it. Therefore, your child's stem cells may not be available after the first year or two. Since a typical pregnancy produces more stem cells than are typically taken by private banks, some families are donating cord blood to both private and public banks. Consult your doctor to help you with this decision.

Embryonic (Blastocyst) Stem Cells

Adult stem cells contain more DNA abnormalities caused by sunlight and environmental and other toxins. Because there is a greater margin for errors when making DNA copies of adult stem cells, scientists have looked to another source of stem cells—those created *in vitro* (outside the body). We'll see in a moment why the term "human embryonic stem cells" (hESC) used by the media is misleading when referring to these *in vitro* cultured cells.

The *in vitro* process is used to assist couples who have difficulty becoming pregnant through the natural method. Let's suppose a couple goes to a lab for fertility assistance. Both partners would donate their reproductive seeds (sperm and ova). The male donates ejaculate material. The female must be heavily sedated while a needle is inserted vaginally to extract eggs from the ovary. The lab successfully fertilizes three eggs for the couple. We now have three zygotes that begin to develop into a morula, then a blastocyst.

A few days after fertilization, the blastocyst is introduced into the woman's uterus and the other two are frozen while the couple waits to see if conception will occur. You may be wondering why the sperm and egg are not frozen separately instead of being united first. A fertilized egg has a much better chance of surviving the freezing process than an unfertilized egg.

The success rate for implantation is about 40% nationwide for women under age thirty-five. If a pregnancy is not achieved, the couple may try again at the appropriate time of the woman's menstrual cycle using another blastocyst they have deposited. Each attempt costs approximately $10,000 to $15,000. Let's say the couple conceives after one try and there are two blastocysts remaining in the lab. Now comes the question, "What would you like the lab to do with the leftover blastocysts?"

The couple presently has four choices:

- Pay to have the cells preserved for another attempt at pregnancy a few years down the road (although the shelf life of a frozen blastocyst is not eternal).

- Simply throw them away if they do not plan to have any more children.

- Let them be used for research in privately-funded labs.

- Give them up for surrogate adoption. A couple with a low sperm count may have the donated blastocyst implanted into their fertile womb and raise the baby as their own.

Many couples actually abandon their leftover blastocysts and leave them at the fertility clinic. In such cases the clinic has no choice but to discard the leftovers.

The field of blastocyst stem cell research is yet to be fully explored due to U.S. government restrictions and the fact that it receives very little public funding due to controversy. Many believe this type of research holds even greater promise than adult stem cells due to the plasticity of the undifferentiated cells.

Ruth R. Faden, Wagley professor of biomedical ethics at Johns Hopkins University, co-wrote an essay with John D. Gearhart, C. Michael Armstrong professor at Johns Hopkins Medicine. Together they report:

> *As much as we might wish it to be otherwise, no non-embryonic sources of stem cells—not stem cells from cord blood or from any "adult" sources—have been shown to have anything like the potential to lead us to viable treatments for such diseases as Juvenile diabetes, Parkinson's and spinal cord injury that stem cells derived from very early embryos do. The science here is unequivocal: Access to embryonic stem cell lines is essential to rapid progress in stem cell research.*[1]

Most scientists believe that research on these stem cells offers the most promise because these stem cells are totipotent, which means they are able to replicate themselves and become any type of cell in the body. Mouse and baboon models prove the concept of "trans-differentiation" or "plasticity" of stem cells—the ability to differentiate into multiple cell types. This is what enables stem cells to replenish themselves and repair tissues in the body. Adult stem cells do not offer the same promise because they are somatic or limited and can only develop into the type of cells found in the organ from which they are taken. Additionally, not all adult organs contain stem cells; therefore not all organs can be regenerated by using adult stem cells. Recent reports show that adult stem cells lose plasticity or shut down to avoid becoming cancerous during the aging process. The mechanisms by which older stem cells shut themselves down was better understood when a gene called *ink4a* was discovered. Ink4a has been found to interfere with the ability of older stem cells to transform into several different types of tissue. This explains why adult stem cells are not adequate to regenerate the parts of the body damaged by Parkinson's or diabetes.

Science does not yet understand how individual parts form during embryogenesis. For example, at a certain stage, the eye looks like a glob of skin cells, but when the tissue behind the eye comes in contact with the skin layer where the eye is going to be, there is an interaction that causes the skin cells to become an eye. We have to understand the chemical conditions, creative signals, and the precise interaction of each and every organ before we can determine why a liver becomes a liver and why a pancreas becomes a pancreas in the embryonic stages of development. There is a huge division of embryology at Vanderbilt University Medical Center that is studying this entire field because it has very important therapeutic implications. Dr. Jagasia states:

"You can't just take a stem cell and unite it with a liver cell

31

or kidney cell and expect it to automatically grow into a new liver. You have to study the conditions and come up with a cocktail of chemicals that are prevalent in the liver or kidney cell and make it look and act like a liver or kidney cell. That will take years and years of research to figure out. Most of the cocktails are available to make a stem cell into a nerve cell or bone marrow cell or a skin cell, but the question is, is that skin cell going to match up with the rest of the skin on the patient's body? Is it going to form a glob or is it going to be smooth, flat skin? With precise technology, we can make a stem cell become a liver cell, but we cannot guarantee that the new liver cell will connect perfectly with the liver cell next to it. What we don't want is a glob of liver cells because that is what we call a tumor. We want a perfectly normal organ. The making of a brain cell from a stem cell has to work in symphony with the cells around it. You can't have a brain cell doing whatever it wants to in one part of the brain or you will have the part of the brain that controls movement, telling an arm or other part of the body to talk.

"Scientists can make frogs with three eyes by manipulating the gene so it receives a signal that cells in a certain place should become an eye. It is not the tissues or mass of cells which will become an eye; it is the interaction of the cells with the skin that will force it to become an eye. The mesoderm is the middle of the three cell layers in an embryo. The visceral organs—the liver, spleen, pancreas, intestines—as well as connective tissue, muscle, blood vessels, bone and muscle and the heart develop from this group of cells. If you look at the vascular system in its early stages, it is just one tube. Why does the tube double up and triple up to become the heart here and stay a tube elsewhere? These are fascinating questions we must be able to answer before we can do embryonic implants on humans. Since we haven't been able to start doing human research, we don't know what the obstacles are. We just don't know what will happen when a manipulated cell is introduced into the human body, and we don't have the funds for the research needed to find out. Even if stem cell research were unlimited today, it would be a couple of decades before we could reach our dream of being able to make a stem cell into a liver and insure that an organized and predictable outcome will be achieved.

"Stem cells are a fascinating group of cells. We can take a patient and blast them with marrow stem cells from a donor at age twenty and have it last a lifetime. If we have been able to perfect that technology using cord blood and bone marrow stem cells to cure cancer and other disorders, there is even more potential with embryonic stem cells that needs to be explored. The hypothesis needs to be tested and it's very likely that if we start testing thirty things, we may get lucky in one.

"Stem cells are very robust and it's tough to manipulate them. They don't like to be poked on or injected and they like certain temperatures and conditions. On one hand they are finicky but on the other they are very strong. When we inject stem cells via bone marrow transplants after using chemo, the patients who survive recover to live normal lives with normal blood counts for the rest of their lives. If we have this type of success using our present technology, you have to believe that using stem cells from blastocysts or embryos would have an even greater potential to expand our ability to cure disease.

"Bone marrow transplant technology was discovered and started being used almost three decades ago. The problem with donor match and recipient rejection remains a problem today, so we are still not 100 percent successful in this technology. If we hadn't had laboratory mice and the ability to play with stem cells thirty or forty years ago, we would not have this technology today. With embryonic stem cells, we've not even reached the starting block.

"If embryonic stem cell research were funded today, it would still need to be in a very controlled environment with ethical, moral, and social investigators with good oversight from protective committees involved. Since there are so many unknowns about this technology, we don't know what to expect. We should start with larger animals. A larger animal is much more similar to a human that a rat is."

Some people believe adult stem cells can be used in the same way as embryonic stem cells, but, as I mentioned earlier, this is not true due to the lack of plasticity of adult cells. Adult stem cells are "fixed" in what they will become and cannot develop into another type of cell. The research done on blastocyst stem cells may very well provide the solution for the shortage of organs needed for those on transplant waiting lists. And the great part is that no one has to die in the process! However, the science is still young and trials on humans have not been completed in every area.

There are still many uncertainties with blastocystic stem cell research that need to be practiced on animals before being introduced to humans. The doors for blastocystic stem cell research in the U.S. are unlocked, but the American government still has its hand on the doorknob. Without federal funds, this area of biological study will not open as quickly or as easily as the research on adult stem cells.

In no way do I suggest we abandon the research and technology for adult stem cells. Instead, the study of blastocyst stem cells should be added to the viable and advanced adult stem cell therapies, which have already proven useful in drug development and for treatment of leukemia, osteopetrosis, heart muscle restoration, and other ailments.

Chapter Two

WHY ALL THE CONTROVERSY?

The medical benefits for humankind are great, and we are on the edge of an era of truly regenerative medical technology. So, why all the controversy? It surely isn't because anyone questions the potential of such research; however, many people question the ethical issues connected with blastocystic stem cells. I propose that the problem is both ignorance and stubbornness. Ignorance about blastocyst stem cell research has caused people to make false assumptions and, even when presented with facts, many are too stubborn to change their mind. As a result, research that very well may produce therapies to aid in health recovery for many people is being hindered.

The main source of controversy arises because some hard-line right-wing religious minorities and anti-abortionist groups believe that harvesting stem cells from *in vitro* fertilization (IVF) procedures destroys an embryo in the process. These groups want you to picture a tiny baby with recognizable arms and legs, little fingers and toes, but, the truth is, IVF eggs are a clump of microscopic cells with no identity. They are not even an organism.

A Matter of Semantics

To give you an idea of why semantics are important to the study of blastocyst cells, I'll give several definitions of terms.

What is an Organism?

Here are four definitions for organism:

- An individual form of life, such as a plant, animal, bacterium, protist (free-living or colonial organisms with diverse nutritional and reproductive modes), or fungus; a body made up of organs, organelles, or other parts that work together to carry on the various processes of life.[2]

- An individual self-sustaining unit of life or living material. Five forms of organisms are known: plants, animals, fungi, protists, and bacteria.[3]

- In biology and ecology, an organism is a living complex adaptive system of organs that influence each other in such a way that they function in some way as a stable whole.[4]

- A living being whose physiological functions are carried out by subunits, or "organs" (like a heart or a liver), which are separate in function but mutually dependent.[5]

By any of these definitions, a blastocyst is not an organism because it does not have a system of organs. It is not self-sustaining and it is not functioning as a whole. Instead, it is totally dependent upon its environment to know what to do next.

A blastocyst is the 32- to 100-cell stage of development reached four to five days after an egg is fertilized. In the blastocyst stage, the inner cell mass that will form the embryo has separated from the cells that will form the placenta, but not all the cells of the inner cell mass will become part of the embryo. Those cells have the same genetic makeup as the embryo cells, yet I don't know of anyone wanting to rescue the other cells. No one has equated the placenta cells of a blastocyst to a human being, so why all the fuss about the rest of the cells of the blastocyst? The blastocyst cannot form an embryo without the placenta.

A blastocyst can only become an organism if it has implanted in a uterus where it receives proper nourishment and signals to differentiate into all the cells and organs required to form a human being.

In light of that knowledge, it is clear that a fish-looking "embryo," as we know it, has not been destroyed in any fertility lab because a fertilized egg is nothing more than a cell cluster. A cell cluster has no nervous system, thus no consciousness. Consciousness is required for humanity to exist.

Terminology is important in any controversial subject— especially when it comes to embryonic stem cell research. So, where did the term come from and why did people start referring to blastocysts as embryos? The ethical arguments regarding the use of human embryos in research date back to 1969 when IVF was first successfully accomplished with a human egg and sperm. The zygotes or blastocysts produced were frozen and stored in fertility clinics for future use. Unfortunately, many people began to call these pending cells "spare embryos." This terminology has created friction between religious anti-abortion groups and those who support blastocyst stem cell research. Once the controversy began, progress with stem cell research on these undifferentiated blastocyst stem cells decreased as the debate increased.

While I don't want to get too fixated on the term "embryo," it is the term that has caused people to take up arms against using stem cells from *in vitro* fertilized eggs for research purposes.

What is an Embryo?

The word embryo originates from the Greek word "embryon," which means "that which grows."[6]

Based on the 2006 Random House Unabridged Dictionary, an embryo is "the young of a mammal, in the early stages of development *within the womb*, in humans up to the end of the second month."[7]

Note: embryo refers to development inside the uterus, not *in vitro*. There are no embryos in a lab dish—there are only cells called zygotes, morulas and blastocysts. There is absolutely no potential for IVF-derived blastocyst stem cells to become a human embryo while in the lab. Mother Nature must do that in the environment of a uterus. To believe otherwise greatly undervalues the woman's role in creating offspring.

Merriam Webster's dictionary defines the term embryo as "an animal in the early stages of growth and differentiation that are characterized by cleavage, the laying down of fundamental tissues, and the formation of primitive organs and organ systems; especially the developing human individual from the time of *implantation* to the end of the eighth week after *conception*."[8]

Note: an embryo has tissues and organs; blastocysts do not. Implantation and conception are considered separate processes and are not synonymous with fertilization.

The American Heritage Dictionary defines embryo as "an organism at any time before full development, birth, or hatching. In humans, the pre-fetal product of conception from implantation through the eighth week of development."[9]

Here, the term embryo is again used to refer to the first two months of development after *conception* confirming that there is a difference between fertilization and conception. That is further confirmed by the fact that an intrauterine device (IUD) does not always prevent fertilization of the egg; it does prevent conception by preventing fertilized eggs (blastocysts) from implanting into the lining of the womb.

Conception and fertilization are two distinct and individual events. While fertilization can occur either in a lab or inside a woman's body, conception can only take place in the womb. Conception occurs when a blastocyst becomes implanted or attached to the lining of the uterus where it begins to receive nourishment for continued development. After the first two months of development inside the womb, the term embryo is replaced by the word "fetus," which applies until birth.

A pregnancy does not actually begin until the process of conception is complete. This process takes several days and can be confirmed by testing the levels of progesterone and hCG (human chorionic gonadotropin) present in the mother's blood. When conception in the uterus is complete, the blastocyst can develop into an embryo. It is very important to remember that conception can only occur inside the uterus.

The American Heritage dictionary gives a second definition for embyro: "an organism in its early developmental stage, before it has a distinctive form; a rudimentary stage." We already know that a blastocyst is not an organism. A lab-created blastocyst is not an embryo; it is no more human than a skin cell, a nerve cell, or any other cell in the human body. If adult stem cells can be used for healing without creating controversy, then why can't *in vitro* blastocyst stem cells be used for research rather than being thrown in the trash?

Harvard's definition of embryo is: "the product of a fertilized egg, from the zygote until the fetal stage." [10] This definition may be the one that provides support for those who say that *in vitro* blastocysts are embryos. Notice that an embryo is the *product* of a fertilized egg—not the fertilized egg itself. Just because the time period from fertilization to 8-weeks of gestation is referred to as embryonic stages, it does not mean that an actual embryo is being formed in the lab. Let's break this down and take a closer look at the definition.

When nature's typical course is followed and *in vitro* procedures are not incorporated, the fertilization of an egg, its implantation into the uterine lining (conception), and the resulting pregnancy is a smooth developmental process that will produce an embryo. But, *in vitro* fertilization is not a process of nature. It is a man-made, scientifically-modified process that unites the sperm and the egg in an environment outside the body. While living cells exist in a blastocyst, the development that must continue in order to carry the cells into fetal stages is not possible unless the blastocyst is introduced to a uterus and nature picks up the cue to begin the process of implantation and subsequent development of an embryo.

Even in the natural process of human reproduction, an embryo does not always develop as a result of fertilization. I am referring to a complete molar pregnancy. This genetic accident occurs when the sperm fertilizes an egg that is either missing its nucleus or where the nucleus is inactive. Even though the egg is fertilized, there is no embryo, no placenta, no fluid, and no amniotic membranes. There is only a mass of cysts that resemble a bunch of grapes. So what does a molar pregnancy have to do with stem cell research? It shows that just because an egg is fertilized, it does not necessarily mean that an embryo has formed.

In one way, doctors and researchers are mislabeling their own product when they refer to fertilized eggs (zygotes, morulas, and blastocysts) as embryonic stem cells. The media is simply repeating this misnomer and fueling the flames of argument. Yes, the cells are within the first two-month stage of development that is covered by the term "embryonic;" however, they are not able to reach all stages of embryonic development until after they successfully implant into the lining of a uterus.

Even though the term "human embryonic stem cell" (hESC) is widely used by the scientific community, I don't like the implication it carries, which suggests that a tiny baby has been formed in the lab. There are better choices for terminology when referring to undifferentiated stem cells created *in vitro*. It might be helpful to call these cells "blastocyst stem cells" or "*in vitro* stem cells." Either of these is a fitting term, which would factually demonstrate that an embryo is not automatically formed when eggs are fertilized *in vitro*. From here on, I will refer to hESC as "IV-B stem cells" unless I am quoting someone who has specifically used the other term. IV-B stands for *in vitro* blastocyst.

I mentioned Reverend Dan Bloodworth in my introduction. While doing his research on stem cells, he was on a video conference call with Dr. Stow and his team of researchers from Cancun, Mexico. Dan told them they had sabotaged their own work by referring to these cells as embryos. "The terminology is misleading and making this a controversial issue it should not be," Dan told them. Their faces showed surprise as the reality sunk in. They had put their work on the "hot" list of anti-abortionist groups who took the term literally and equated it with abortion. After all, the destruction or removal of an embryo from the womb is considered an abortion. Since embryos are not removed from the womb in any fertility lab, research on, or even the disposal of, *in vitro* blastocysts cannot be equated to abortion or the loss of human life. The development of an embryo has not even begun; therefore, it is not ended.

What is a Fetus?

By the eighth week of gestation (which must take place inside the uterus), organs have begun to develop and the heart is beating. Remember that, in humans, the term "fetus" refers to stages of development two months or longer; thus, the correct term to use after eight weeks is fetus, not embryo. I am neither for nor against abortion of an embryo. A flower is only a weed if it exists where a human does not want it. I suppose it is the same with an unwanted pregnancy. An embryo in its early stages does not have a brain, nerve function, or heart beat. I feel that each situation has to be examined individually, and a decision must be made based upon the highest and best for each person involved. I can't say whether it is murder for a woman to terminate a pregnancy if her life is in danger, or if she is mentally, financially, or emotionally unable to care for a child, or if she has become pregnant as a result of rape or incest, or while using birth control. We each live with the consequences of our own decisions, and we are not called to judge one another.

IV-B stem cells never will develop into a baby unless the entire blastocyst is implanted into a uterus—either of the female who donated the egg or that of a surrogate mother. Let me clarify that the stem cells used for blastocyst research purposes are only a few days old and have *never* been inside a uterus. These cells are not equal to a human life. They have no nerve or blood cells; they have no consciousness. Research conducted in university laboratories in partnership with Geron Corporation supports the fact that IVF-derived blastocyst stem cells are not embryos because they are not a complete organism, nor can they be coaxed into becoming such outside the uterus.

The inner cell mass of a blastocyst contains pluripotent stem cells, which have the ability to form any of the more than 260 types of cells of a human body. At this point of development the father's DNA and the mother's DNA are present, but the entity it would stand to create has no identity. The morula or blastocyst cells are undefined, which means that under certain conditions they could become tissue, cells, organs, blood vessels, or, if unhindered in the natural environment of the womb, they could develop into a human being. However, at the point in which these cells are used for research (4-5 days), they have not taken the form of a human being. Similar to the seed of a plant having the ability to become a mature plant, the life force contained in these undifferentiated cells has the potential to become anything if the conditions are suitable for such development. An *in vitro* fertilized egg is no more a human being than an acorn is an oak tree.

The *in vitro* process is used to help a woman bear a child, but the extra cells that are not going to be implanted can also be used to become cells, tissues, or organs that offer hope, or possibly a cure, for someone who suffers from disease or injury. Either option benefits humankind! Discarding unused blastocysts serves no purpose at all.

What are the Ethical Issues Involved?

Using human material in research is an issue of contention because it has been misconstrued as the sacrifice of human life for scientific progress. My question to those who object to all IV-B stem cell research on the basis of the sanctity of life is this: Why is it less moral to use these cells for research than it is to destroy them? Blastocysts leftover from *in vitro* fertilization that are not "adopted" for surrogacy are placed into a plastic medical waste container and discarded as medical garbage.

The Clinton Administration argued that funding for human blastocystic research was an appropriate government function due to its therapeutic abilities already proven. However, the Clinton Administration came to an end before the law was changed; and no funding was provided. President George W. Bush vetoed The Stem Cell Research Enhancement Act (H.R. 810) to expand blastocyst stem cell research in July 2006 because, in his words, "It crosses a moral boundary that our decent society needs to respect." This legislation, which passed both houses of Congress with significant bipartisan support, would have expanded the number of blastocyst stem cell cultures eligible for federally funded research.

On August 12, 2001, President Bush said:

> *Stem cell research is still at an early, uncertain stage, but the hope it offers is amazing: infinitely adaptable human cells to replace damaged or defective tissue and treat a wide variety of diseases. Yet the ethics of medicine are not infinitely adaptable. There is at least one bright line: We do not end some lives for the medical benefit of others. For me, this is a matter of conviction: a belief that life, including early life, is biologically human, genetically distinct and valuable.*[11]

My question is: if blastocyst stem cells are so genetically distinct and biologically *human,* why are these cells able to benefit rats? Since the 1980s, researchers have been experimenting with blastocystic stem cells in mice. Dr. Evan Snyder was part of a

Harvard research team that took neural stem cells from the brain of a human fetus, cloned new cells exactly like them, and injected the cultured cells into the brains of developing mice. These cells made their way to various parts of the brain, developed into the correct types of brain cells, integrated successfully with cells in other parts of the brain, and took on characteristics and functions that would normally take place during development of a mouse brain. The mice showed restored movement and lived longer lives than those mice having the same problem that were not treated. Since rodents have the same kinds of cells as humans, it is reasonable to believe that this transplant technology could re-grow nerves in the spinal cord of humans. I never thought I would be thanking a rat, but these little creatures are sacrificing more for this research than any of us!

When Does Life Begin?

Some critics uphold the notion that the *in vitro* process creates an embryo, and that human life should not be created for medical or scientific purposes. The process of stem cell research starts with living cells (ova and sperm) and ends with living cells. No life or death has occurred in the process. The cells scientists want to use for research are the leftover IV-Bs. No one is suggesting that IVF be used to create blastocysts specifically for use in research. Give them funding to use the ones already headed for the biohazard containers. Let them find a way to help the living, breathing human beings who are suffering.

I propose that there is no real beginning or ending of life. Bear with me while I explain my metaphysical understanding of this topic. We are spirit beings occupying human flesh. Everything on this planet has life force (primordial energy or creative force) or it could not exist. There is no such thing as a "non-living" object because without the life force, there is no change, growth, or development—not even in a stone that takes millions of years to change its structure! When an animal, human or plant dies the process of decay immediately begins. Decomposition is an enzymatic process where living cells break down molecules and atoms and change them into something else—soil or earth, which then contains the life force to nurture a seed or plant. Life and death are part of a cycle.

The one factor that spawns the most controversy in abortion issues and blastocystic stem cell technology is "When does life begin?" I personally believe that life begins before fertilization because the egg and the sperm are living cells. However, the determination of the "origination of human life" is where the battle lies in determining whether a life is being sacrificed if the growth process is terminated at a particular stage of development. Even though there is no real way to prove when human life begins, I must address this point and evaluate the possibilities. I'll begin with a source of reference many Americans are familiar with—the Bible. The Bible says in Genesis 2:7, "The Lord God formed the man from the dust of the ground and breathed into his nostrils the breath of life, and the man became a living soul." If you believe that, then surely you are not the one creating controversy about conducting research on cells that aren't breathing. Based on this verse, a fetus that is sucking its thumb and kicking its mother's bladder is not a living soul because it is not breathing. I doubt there are many people who literally believe that life does not begin until a baby is born and takes its first breath.

Some people say life begins when an egg is fertilized. Others believe it begins when conception occurs or when the fertilized egg implants itself into the lining of the womb and begins to draw nourishment from the mother. Prior to the late 19th century, theologians believed the soul entered its human host at "quickening," which may be felt by the mother approximately twenty weeks after conception.

According to Rabbi Elliot Dorff, a scholar in Judaism and medical ethics issues, the Hebrew Talmud states that an embryo based on the definitions of gestation, are considered "like water until the 40th day." Rabbi Dorff further explains, "According to the Jewish view, this genetic material outside the uterus has no chance of developing into a human being unless transplanted into a woman. As such, it has even less legal status in Judaism than zygotes and embryos in the womb...unlike the Catholic Church, we don't consider this genetic material to have a soul or to be a human being, or to even have the status of potentially being a life.[12]

Reverend Dan and Carol Bloodworth's adult son, Brian, is in a stage 4 coma and is fed through a tube. He has been unable to do a thing for himself since he was struck by lightning as a junior in high school. Reverend Bloodworth has been lobbying for stem cell research for more than 16 years in hopes of finding help for his son. As a result of his extensive knowledge on the topic, Dan has been appointed to the Advisory Council to Congress regarding stem cell research. Even though Dan and I disagree in our theology (I endorse a metaphysical view of life; Dan is an all-denominational evangelist) our hearts are knit as we focus on those things we have in common. Those things are our love for humanity, our belief in a Divine Creator, and our desire to see all types of stem cell research federally funded. I value Dan's opinion and the research he has done on this topic. Therefore, I will refer to him throughout this book. In fact, the next chapter will present his Biblical support for blastocyst stem cell research.

Dan Bloodworth's mission is to lift people up and help them anyway he can. In doing so, he is following in his father's footsteps. Elvis Bloodworth only had an eighth grade education, but he taught rheumatology to doctors at Vanderbilt University. He had a reason to find out all that he could about rheumatology because he suffered with rheumatoid arthritis. He completed years of research and held the ear of 26 doctors who were studying this field. The elder Bloodworth allowed his living body to be used as a human guinea pig to seek a cure for rheumatoid arthritis. He participated in experimental programs at the Mayo Clinic, Walter Reed Hospital, and in research centers in Mexico. Complications from some experimental drugs caused his ribs to perforate and cave in on his heart where it caused muscle and valve damage. He was facing heart surgery to repair the damage when Vanderbilt University Medical Center (VUMC), Baptist Hospital, and St. Thomas Hospital joined as a team to do an experimental surgery on Elvis to completely rebuild a new ribcage for him made from synthetic material. Elvis was in surgery for over thirteen hours, and there were complications causing Bloodworth to die on the table two times. Surgeons were able to revive him and he lived four more years.

Dan made a statement at his father's funeral, "I'll walk in my dad's footsteps, but I'll never fill his shoes." About a year ago his sister said of Dan, "He said he would never fill our dad's shoes, but he has done exactly that. He has done for stem cell research what our father did for rheumatoid arthritis—educate the world with scientific facts."

When Dan realized that Bible-believing fundamentalist

conservatives are the main group of people who oppose blastocyst stem cell research, he went to Rhema Bible College to better understand their logic. According to Dan, the Bible mentions the word "blood" 499 times, making it the second most important subject in the Bible—the first of which is "love." The Bible states in Leviticus 17, verses 11 and 14 that "The life of a creature is in the blood....you must not eat the blood of any creature, because the life of every creature is its blood." If that is true, then a fertilized egg is not alive because it does not contain blood.

According to Dr. John Gearhart of Johns Hopkins Medical Center, Dr. Evan Snyder of Burnham Institute, and other researchers in the field of embryonic development, the formation of blood cells and blood vessels start at the beginning of the third week after fertilization, first in the yolk sac and outer membrane surrounding the embryo. About two days later, blood vessels begin to form in the embryo body. However, blood is not formed in the embryo body until the fifth week. So, according to the Bible and the science of embryology, we are safe to assume that we are not taking a life if we terminate the growth of embryonic cells prior to the third week of development. Some Christians believe the Leviticus verses refer to the blood of Jesus Christ. That is not possible. The Old Testament is a Jewish book written long before Jesus was ever born.

When Reverend Bloodworth travels the country and speaks of this verse, preachers and parishioners are astounded because they simply did not know that fertilized eggs do not have blood in them. They are still seeing the little miniature baby swimming around in its mother's womb. They have never been given factual or scientific information about blastocyst stem cells, and they haven't done any research on their own. Instead, they are willing to naively believe other people who have told them that IV-B stem cell research kills babies.

When anti-stem cell crusaders say that they oppose stem cell research because of moral and ethical aspects, there is rarely any mention of biology or any scientific foundation for their moral conclusions. Dan's wife, Carol, is the television director for Trinity Broadcasting Network in Nashville, Tennessee; therefore, Dan has contact with a lot of evangelists who appear as guests on the show. When Dan approaches them about their stance on stem cell research, he asks them what they are basing their facts on. They can only give their opinion, which was probably handed to them by someone else. When Dan shares the facts about there not being blood in the cells and gives Bible verses that support stem cell research, they are dumbfounded. Not one of them has ever given him one verse of scripture that backs up their opinion.

Many times these preachers have a large following of people who believe every word they say is from God. Ignorance about stem cell research has given some religious leaders a lot of power over their followers. Many a person will tithe their last dollar to keep their religious leader wearing silk suits and will stand in line to cast a vote to help put their hero in office. Religious and political leaders have a serious obligation to research and find out whether or not what they are telling people is true.

Stem cell biologist, Dr. John A. Kessler wrote an essay titled "I want to see my daughter walk again," which was published by Chicago Tribune June 13, 2004. Dr. Kessler's daughter suffered a spinal-cord injury in a skiing accident and is confined to a wheelchair. What upsets him the most about the stem cell controversy are the people who impose personal beliefs on the rest of the world in an effort to prevent research that might help his daughter and others like her who have an incurable malady that might one day be treatable with stem-cell therapies.

There is also rarely any discussion of biology or any scientific rationale for their moral judgments. Their opposition to stem cell research focuses primarily on two issues: the process of somatic cell nuclear transfer (therapeutic cloning) and the use by researchers of frozen embryos that are otherwise slated to be destroyed.

It is important to keep in mind that we are discussing a microscopic cluster of no more than 200 cells that has absolutely no potential to develop into a human being unless it is implanted in a uterus. The profound difference between fertilization and conception is frequently forgotten. Fertilization can happen in a laboratory, but the conception of a human individual can only happen after the fertilized oocyte is implanted in the uterus.

The moral obligation to help other human beings is a concept universal to virtually all religions, and the entire focus of stem-cell biology is on alleviating human suffering and disease. Anti-stem-cell crusaders seem to place more importance on a cluster of cells that has no possibility of becoming a human than on the suffering and needs of real human beings.[13]

Now, we've heard it from a preacher and a scientist that the ones in opposition to blastocyst stem cell research rarely have any good support for their opinion.

Get this: an *opinion* that cannot be supported by scientific fact or scripture is preventing funding for a technology that quite possibly holds salvation for millions in our world who are suffering. Those in opposition have no basis for believing that using stem cells derived from 3- to 5-day-old fertilized eggs grown in a laboratory are human beings. By now you realize that you have been fed a lie based upon someone's opinion or assumption. Perhaps you are ready to accept that blastocyst stem cells leftover from IVF procedures should be used for research.

The arguments about blastocyst stem cell research have been ongoing for thirty years. Shortly after the Supreme Court rendered its decision on Roe versus Wade in 1973, which legalized abortion nationwide, research on the cells of aborted fetuses has not been funded by the U.S. Government. A constitutional moratorium was enacted that banned federal funding for clinical research on "a living human fetus, before or after the induced abortion of such fetus, unless such research is done for the purpose of assuring the survival of such fetus." The moratorium was a temporary measure to give Congress time to set up a National Commission for the Protection of Human Subjects of Biomedical and Behavioral Research responsible for offering guidelines on human fetal and embryo research. The Commission was aware of the possible uses of embryos. The moratorium was lifted in 1975 when the Commission voted to temporarily establish a National Ethics Advisory Board to review proposed standards and research protocols for federal funding of embryonic research. In 1978, human IVF techniques produced a live-born child after fertilized eggs were introduced into the uterus of a woman. As a result, IVF research and human fetal research were identified as two separate issues. The Ethics Advisory Board agreed that it would be ethical to allow federal funding for research provided the research did not take place on embryos beyond fourteen days of development and that all donors were married couples (as if marital status has something to do with the technology).

The Department of Health, Education and Welfare (DHEW, the precursor to today's Department of Health and Human Services) decided to offer funding for IVF but not for human embryo studies on aborted fetuses. This decision has remained in effect because the Ethics Advisory Board's charter expired in 1980 and was not replaced or renewed. The Stem Cell Research Enhancement Act, H.R. 3 was passed by the House of Representatives in January 2007. It was again passed (as Senate bill 5) through Congress 63 to 37 in April 2007. This bill would help America maintain (or regain) a leadership role in the global field of science and medicine by allowing scientists to use IV-Bs created after August 2001. However, President Bush has vowed to veto it a second time as he caters to the minority of voices who oppose it.

Through the National Institutions of Health (NIH) Revitalization Act in 1993, Congress cancelled the requirement that research etiquette be approved by the Ethics Advisory Board which had not existed for 13 years. A Human Embryo Research Panel was called forth to consider the issues regarding human embryo research and to offer standards for potential funding applications. Some areas of human embryo research were deemed eligible for federal funding providing certain ethical safeguards were adhered to. The 1996 Departments of Labor, Health and Human Services and Education, and Related Agencies Appropriations Act (also known as the Dickey Amendment) prohibits the use of any federal funds for research that destroys or seriously endangers human embryos, or creates them for research purposes. However, the Bush Administration's interpretation of the Dickey Amendment allows funding of research using blastocysts left over from IVF procedures provided they were created prior to August 9, 2001.

When research at the University of Wisconsin, supported by private funds from the Geron Corporation and the University's Alumni Research Foundation, began to show significantly promising technology on stem cells, people began to reconsider federal funding for IV-B stem cell research. Most members of Congress and supporters of the Dickey Amendment still believe nascent human life ought to be protected against exploitation and destruction for scientific purposes and, to this day, is not supported by taxpayer dollars.

A blastocyst is not necessarily destroyed when stem cells are taken from it. Biologists can take a single cell from a blastocyst, study the DNA (pre-implantation genetics) and determine its health and other characteristics without harming it. For example, if a couple desires to have a child, but one partner has cystic fibrosis, they can have their fertilized egg (blastocyst) examined before it is implanted into the womb to make sure it is free of the cystic fibrosis gene. A healthy blastocyst would then be implanted rather than one having the diseased gene. This technology has been perfected to the extent that if you take one cell out of the inner cell mass of the blastocyst it does not affect the blastocyst as it comes into the embryo and fetal stages of development. You could potentially take a cell from a blastocyst and coax it into growing more undifferentiated stem cells without harming the remaining blastocyst.

If the U.S. is willing to fund research on a limited number of IV-B stem cells and unwilling to fund research done on embryos/fetuses, there should be distinction between the two types of research. It is not fair to say that *all* research done prior to birth is equal to abortion. Abortion has to do with the removal of an embryo or fetus from the womb. Research using IV-B stem cells does not terminate a pregnancy because no pregnancy has occurred in the lab dish.

When the Bush Administration looked at the policy regarding blastocyst stem cell research in 2001, the regulations proposed by the Clinton Administration were put on hold until they could be further reviewed. The Bush Administration dumped Clinton's Bioethics Council and approved his own council directed by an opponent of IV-B stem cell research, Leon Kass.

While continuing to withhold taxpayer support for research on blastocysts, the Bush Administration decided to allow IVF-derived blastocyst stem cell research on approximately sixty lines created prior to August 9, 2001, because their fate had already been decided within the measure of the law. I might add that since both abortion and IVF are both legal procedures, the fate of *all* aborted embryos/fetuses and unused IV-B stem cells has also been decided, and there is really no reason to fund one and not the other.

President Bush's policy has been contested ever since its announcement, not only by those who contend the moral, legal, and political implications are too liberal, but also by researchers, physicians, and patient advocacy groups who believe the guidelines are too restrictive and frustrate the growth of a very important area of research. While some are concerned that it is unethical to disrupt the development of fertilized eggs, I think the real question is "Is it ethical to withhold support and funding for a research that holds such human promise?"

What Defines Death Anyway?

When does a human being die? Is it when the heart stops beating or when the lungs stop breathing? A person can be kept alive with machines, and most people agree that as long as a person has brain waves, they are still "technically" alive. When does a blastocyst die? Blastocysts have no heart, lungs, nerves or brain.

Most people don't have a problem killing and eating an animal to nourish human life, but many can't seem to remove the issue of death regarding human eggs in a lab dish.

For the sake of playing devil's advocate, let's entertain the notion that a 3- to 5-day old fertilized egg is actually a human life. Isn't it a Christian belief that it is okay to sacrifice the life of one for the good of many? Wasn't Jesus' life sacrificed in order that many could be saved? Why couldn't a few martyred cells be used to save the lives of millions who are lost and without hope for healing? What would Jesus do? As a healer, he would be an advocate for all types of stem cell research.

Not All Seeds are Destined for Maturity

Looking at nature, we see that not every fertilized egg or sprouted seed (nascent life) was meant to make it to full term. In Matthew 13:3-8 of the Bible we read:

> *Then he (Jesus) told them many things in parables, saying, "A farmer went out to sow his seed. As he was scattering the seed, some fell along the path, and the birds came and ate it up. Some fell on rocky places, where it did not have much soil. It sprang up quickly, because the soil was shallow. But when the sun came up, the plants were scorched, and they withered because they had no root. Other seed fell among thorns, which grew up and choked the plants. Still other seed fell on good soil, where it produced a crop—a hundred, sixty or thirty times what was sown."*

From this we gather that only 25 percent of the seeds sown actually make it to maturity. Some are used to nourish other forms of life (birds). It's the same with human seeds (eggs). Not all eggs ripened in the ovary will be fertilized. Not all fertilized eggs will implant into a uterus. Not all blastocysts will develop into embryos. Not all embryos will become fetuses; some fetuses will miscarry; some will be born to live only a short while after birth, while others will be born and live a long life as an adult. Similar to the seed of a plant, the life force contained in blastocyst stem cells has the potential to advance to the next stage if conditions are suitable. Why not allow the cells left over from *in vitro* fertilization to become something that offers hope, or possibly a cure, for those who suffer from disease and injury?

I promise you, the American Government is not really worried about the moral status of human embryos. After all, it does allow abortion. The NIH guidelines published in 2000 and the decision made by the Bush Administration in 2001 show that the U.S. government is in favor of research on blastocyst stem cells, as long as it is done with private funds rather than with the taxpayer's dollar. Federal funds may be used on a few stem cell lines from leftover *in vitro* processes. So, is this really the moral issue our politicians pretend it to be?

IVF processes are used to help a woman bear a child, but the extra cells that are not going to be implanted can also be used to help others. Once scientists learn how these cells become tissues or organs these cells may offer hope, or possibly a cure, for someone who suffers from disease or injury. What a benefit to humankind! Discarding unused blastocysts serves no purpose at all.

Why are some Americans on a crusade to save the cells? By withholding federal funds from blastocyst stem cell research, progress toward many cures is being hindered. Rather than worrying about cells in a lab dish that will never become a human being, there should be some accountability for the real human lives lost. Shouldn't those in opposition to the research be held responsible for murder of those who might have been cured? Those suffering are our friends, family members, and neighbors with whom we have a relationship.

Chapter Three

BIBLICAL SUPPORT FOR BLASTOCYSTIC RESEARCH

I want to distinguish between people of faith and the ultra-conservative "religious right." People of faith are open-minded individuals who embrace their own spirituality without trying to force their beliefs on others. They are not inclined to react with prejudice toward others. It is for the people of faith that I write this book.

Members of the religious right are strong-willed, dogma-driven, and intolerant of those who disagree with them. They tend to be illogical regarding social standards and are not likely to be convinced that they are doing harm by preventing blastocyst stem cell research from moving forward. They use their religious beliefs to fight scientific progress no matter what facts are presented to them.

People of faith truly want to learn more about blastocyst stem cell research in order to form an intelligent opinion of their own. Perhaps that's why you are reading this book. Regardless of what "brand" of faith you hold, or even if you have no affiliation with any religious group, I believe you will find this Biblical information helpful.

RIGHT TO RECOVER—*Yvonne Perry*

After Reverend Dan Bloodworth shared his findings and Biblically supportive information with Former Republican Leader Senator Bill Frist of Tennessee, Senator Frist became a major supporter of federal financing for blastocystic stem cell research. He even spoke against President Bush's veto of H.R. 810 in July 2006, which would have allowed research on stem cell lines previously frozen for use in fertility treatments. When Dan told a group of nuns who were anti-abortion advocates he was against abortion, they were shocked. They thought he had to be pro-abortion if he supported IV-B research. Once he shared his scientific and Biblical findings on blastocyst stem cell research, all the nuns realized they had been misled to believe that blastocystic stem cell research equated to abortion. All of the nuns, except for Mother Superior, hugged Dan or shook his hand and thanked him for showing them that even the Pope could be wrong—even though he is supposed to be divinely taught.

Reverend Bloodworth attended Rhema Bible College in order to better understand how the right wing beliefs were supported. His education led him to believe that stem cell research and any subsequent therapy is a gift from God, and showed him that the logic of those who oppose IV-B stem cell research is unfounded. Neither the scripture nor biological data can be used to support that a life is being taken when blastocyst stem cells are used for research. I'm sure you would like to know what Reverend Bloodworth shared that was so convincing. Here are his findings:

Stem cell research of any kind is of God, not against God. According to John 1:3, all things are created by God and without Him nothing has been created that was created. The science of stem cell technology is created by God.

Hosea 4:6

> *My people are destroyed from lack of knowledge. Because you have rejected knowledge, I also reject you as my priests; because you have ignored the law of your God, I also will ignore your children.*

Ignorance is not bliss; it's dangerous!

Malachi 3:6

> *"I, the LORD, do not change. So you, O descendants of Jacob, are not destroyed."*

If God cannot change, and we need blood to be born the second time (salvation through the blood of Jesus Christ), then we can't be born without blood the first time.

John 1:13 New International Version

> *Children born not of natural descent, nor of human decision or a husband's will, but born of God. (NIV)*

> *Not of the flesh, not of human desire, nor of the blood but of the Holy Spirit. (KJV)*

In other words, neither the fleshly act (coitus) nor the desire to get pregnant, and not even the appearance of blood guarantees that life will begin. Life only comes if the Holy Spirit deems it to be. Some time after blood appears, the Holy Spirit enters the womb and purposes whether or not the potential life is to become a live human baby. The blood must be present before this takes place. Remember, God is always the same. He doesn't do things one way one time and another way the next.

John 6:62-65:

> ...*The Spirit gives life; the flesh counts for nothing. The words I have spoken to you are spirit and they are life. Yet there are some of you who do not believe. For Jesus had known from the beginning which of them did not believe and who would betray him. He went on to say, "This is why I told you that no one can come to me unless the Father has enabled him."*

God gives life, not the body. Humans look at the flesh and not at the spirit, which gives life.

I Corinthians 2:4-5

> *My message and my preaching were not with wise and persuasive words, but with a demonstration of the Spirit's power, so that your faith might not rest on men's wisdom, but on God's power.*

God always shows us an example of his greatness and the way he wants us to go. Notice he stated not to rely on man's wisdom alone.

I Corinthians 3:9-11

> *For we are God's fellow workers; you are God's field, God's building. By the grace God has given me, I laid a foundation as an expert builder, and someone else is building on it. But each one should be careful how he builds. For no one can lay any foundation other than the one already laid, which is Jesus Christ.*

We are God's fellow workers. Stem cell technology used to create healing is part of God's perfect plan, and we have the privilege to carefully use the knowledge and abilities he gives us. As with any power, it can be misused and abused. To not use this technology to help others would be a great abuse of power. The Good Samaritan would do whatever it took to help others. It would be like leaving the beggar in the ditch and passing by on our self-righteous way. What would Jesus do? I assure you he wouldn't even leave an ox in the ditch on the Sabbath. He healed everyone who asked him.

Ephesians 3:20

Now to him who is able to do immeasurably more than all we ask or imagine, according to his power that is at work within us.

Ephesians 2:10

For we are God's workmanship, created in Christ Jesus to do good works, which God prepared in advance for us to do.

These verses imply that God works through humans, and that without our cooperation He accomplishes nothing on Earth. All knowledge, skills, talents, and capabilities are representative of God's power working through us. God planned for stem cell technology to work as a healing tool, but we must allow this good work.

According to the 2002 U.S. Census data, eighteen percent of our population is suffering from debilitating diseases. Jesus isn't coming back for a sick church! God is trying to get the body of Christ well. Church leadership is running from new technologies instead of embracing and understanding what God is trying to accomplish through them.

RIGHT TO RECOVER—*Yvonne Perry*

James 1:17

> *Every good gift and every perfect gift is from above, and cometh down from the Father of lights, with whom is no variableness, neither shadow of turning.*

Stem cell technology, in the limited way we know it now, is a great gift for, and to, humankind. The future of IV-B technology is even greater. Imagine being on the donor list and being able to receive a heart without another person having to die in order to donate it. The heart and other organs may be created in a laboratory one day. Where do good gifts come from? How faithful will we be to use our God-given skills, abilities, and gifts to help others?

***

I didn't attend church for 40 years without learning something about the Bible, so here is my own input using Scripture.

John 12:24

> *I tell you the truth, unless a kernel of wheat falls to the ground and dies, it remains only a single seed. But if it dies, it produces many seeds.*

My grandmother and I (Yvonne) raised a garden together for many years. When we were planting the seeds each spring, she would always remind me to plant four seeds to each hole we dug: two for the birds, one for the weather, and one for us. Even with our generous planting regime, we nearly always had to replant a second time to fill in the holes where none of the seeds survived.

Going back to nature, let's compare a plant seed to a fertilized egg. Both a seed and a zygote hold the potential for reproducing life. When a seed is planted into the ground, it begins to draw nourishment from the soil. This can be considered the conception or beginning of life. It is the same with a fertilized egg. It must be implanted in a woman's womb in order to become an organism. From this, we see that fertilization and conception are not synonymous and do not occur at the same time.

In order to determine whether we are talking about the beginning of cell division or the beginning of a pregnancy, we need to be reminded of the difference between fertilization and conception.

Fertilization of a human egg may occur in the fallopian tube or *in vitro* by scientific means. It takes only a few hours after the sperm and ovum unite to start the process of cell division.

Conception occurs when a fertilized egg, which has become a blastocyst, implants itself into the uterine lining and begins to draw nourishment from the mother. This can be confirmed by testing hCG levels.

Thus, we correctly use the term "*in vitro* fertilization" but not "*in vitro* conception." Be aware of the indispensable role of a woman in childbirth. Without a mother's womb, there is no baby.

"Ignorant preachers and teachers have not done their research," says Dan Bloodworth. "People, all too willingly follow a person rather than their inner voice or intuition, and are quick to jump on the bandwagon, even if the wagon is going to destroy someone's chances for recovery."

Right-wing ultra-conservatives are destroying their own platform and decreasing the following they have built for themselves. Sermon after righteous sermon, these people have been telling everyone else what to do, how to do it, what's right, what's sinful, but then the truth comes out. Their hypocritical actions reveal to us that those we have put on a pedestal are as guilty as the ones they condemn. And these people tell us that blastocyst stem cell research is equal to murder. Can we trust anything they say? It's no wonder fewer and fewer people are adhering to the traditional belief systems passed to them by family, society, and religious leaders.

Neoconservatives

The religious right's opposition to blastocystic stem cell research lies primarily within the neoconservative movement. The term neoconservatism stems from Eric Voegelin (*Order and History*) and Leo Strauss *(Natural Right and History)*—two confrontational political philosophers who believe religion in the government is necessary to keep order (control) in society. Strauss's and Voegelin's books were written shortly after World War II and soon had a following. This communistic view was further developed by Irving Kristol and carried on by his son William Kristol.

Neoconservatives have taken into their ranks other groups who are against anything that is pleasurable or that allows one the freedom to enjoy life. With an emphasis on original sin and the body being "unclean," these wrathful ideas found their way into the doctrine of America's mainstream denominations. Dictatorial characteristics are seen in the bitter leadership of ultra-orthodox Catholic and Christian fundamentalist religions that oppose free-thinking liberalist ideas and attack homosexuals, pro-abortionists, and anyone who doesn't fit their mold or live by their moral code. They are also against science and keep a steady discourse debating its worth. Kristol admitted that he did not believe in the religious "myths" that portray God as a ruthless and angry deity that must be obeyed, but he felt it necessary for people to be afraid of the "powers that be" in order to maintain unity in society.

Opus Dei (O.D.) is one of the exclusionary groups that adheres to this offensive and condemning philosophy that values war and killing as a means to attaining world order. Members seek personal Christian perfection, strive to implement Christian ideals in their chosen occupations, and promote Christian values to society as a whole. U.S. Senators Sam Brownback (R-KS) and Rick Santorum (R-PA) and U.S. Supreme Court Justice Clarence Thomas are some of the most outspoken opponents to blastocyst stem cell research. While they have not claimed to be members of Opus Dei, their behavior fits the definition of O.D. cooperator: to help the apostolates of the Prelature aimed at promoting at all levels of society the universal call to sanctity, especially through the sanctification of ordinary work and of family life.[14]

Eric Cohen strongly supported President Bush's invasion of Iraq. Mr. Cohen and the three men mentioned above adamantly oppose blastocystic stem cell research. Cohen admits that cures will come from the research and believes that medical breakthroughs will result.

In an article titled "Neoconning the Media, A Very Short History of Neoconservatism" Eric Alterman, weblogger for MSNBC.com, wrote about Mr. Cohen:

> *Mr. Cohen sees nothing hypocritical about sending natural born Americans to die in an ill-chosen battle in what is supposed to be a war on terrorism, but finds revulsion in using spare embryos destined for destruction to be used to heal the sick and disabled. Straussian neoconservatives constantly celebrate in their writings virtue in war, as if peace were sinful.*

…Their war on Iraq has proven a catastrophe by almost any available measure but they are already planning another adventure in Iran. …The United States is now less safe, poorer, more hated and more constrained in its ability to fight terrorism than it was before the tragic loss of blood and treasure the war has demanded. And yet the Neocons have admitted almost no mistakes and continue to be rewarded with plum posts in the Bush Administration.[15]

Frank Cocozzelli

Next, I'd like to present to you a perspective by Frank L. Cocozzelli of the Institute for Progressive Christianity. Frank is the author of *"By the Better Angels of Our Nature,"* which is a plan of action to revive centrist liberalism. Mr. Cocozzelli is a private practice New York City attorney afflicted with muscular dystrophy. He is a political advocate for expanded blastocystic stem cell research that could conceivably help him walk again. As a liberal Catholic, Frank speaks on issues of progressive faith.

When Pope Benedict XVI voiced opposition to blastocystic stem cell research by using Psalm 39 to support his belief that an embryo is equivalent to a natural born human being, Cocozzelli replied in an article on Talk2Action titled *Neoconservatism, the Catholic Church and Stem Cells*:

However, this contention is not universally accepted by the many who practice one of the various Judeo-Christian faiths— including a clear majority of American Catholics. I am one of those Church-going Roman Catholics who cannot accept such an interpretation…

Scripture alone would appear to refute the Pontiff's interpretation, particularly, Jeremiah, 1:15 which states: "Before I formed you in the belly, I knew you. Before you came forth out of the womb, I sanctified you. I have appointed you a prophet to the nations." This would imply that an individual first needs to be a fetus, not merely an embryo before personhood exists. And by any way biology is approached, a womb is still needed to transform an embryo into a fetus: it is an irrefutable requirement.

But for me as Catholic, I find myself seeking the position Jesus would take. The Gospels consistently detail His adherence to pekuach nefesh* through His many acts of healing. And as a Catholic who has read the Gospels, I cannot recall Jesus directly refuting pekuach nefesh. It logically follows that a Jesus who lived by Jewish law raises a presumption that He would not oppose this vital medical research. If anything, His healing the infirmed and disabled along with raising the dead for me is what contradicts the Pontiff's position.[16]

All I can say to that is, "Amen, Brother Frank!"

Now that we've had a science class and a Sunday school lesson, let's see how we can best incorporate this knowledge.

- Stop following the crowd!

- Do your own research and form your own opinion using scientific facts. A guilty conscious is emotionally subject to the opinions of others. Decide with your logical mind.

- Then, share with others what you have learned.

Whether you claim to be a Christian or an Atheist, you can confidently support blastocystic stem cell research. It does not harm nascent life. It will help us work together for the common good of all people on this planet. Isn't that what being a good, global citizen is all about?

*The law of pekuach nefesh REQUIRES that almost all Jewish law MUST be violated if necessary to save a life.

Chapter Four

SEPARATION OF CHURCH AND STATE

Now that we have shown Biblical support for science and medicine, we see that all stem cell research is a gift that holds the keys to restoring health. Since God is not willing that any of us should perish, we can begin to turn away from any preconceived notion that withholds the blessing of health from ourselves and others. Next, I'd like to investigate how religion came to influence so many of our decisions including the governing of our country.

While I do not intend any derogatory comments about our government or our religious community, there are certain facts and issues that must be addressed in order to educate and help readers understand the impact that religion and politics have upon our society. I suppose the best place to begin is with the founding of our country.

You may not realize it, but America was not founded upon Christianity. That may be what you were taught in school, but proof of such is not reflected in the writings of our founding fathers. Evangelist Billy Graham agrees that the United States of America is not a Christian nation. In a televised interview on

RIGHT TO RECOVER—*Yvonne Perry*

May 30, 1997, David Frost asked Mr. Graham, "Say, is this still a Christian Country?" To which Billy Graham replied, "No! We're not a Christian Country. We've never been a Christian Country. We're a secular Country, by our Constitution. In which Christians live and which many Christians have a voice. But we're not a Christian Country.[17]

In fact, the first six American presidents and many notable founding fathers were actually opposed to Christianity. Hard to believe isn't it? Let me give some examples.

Known as the "Father of our Country," President George Washington (1789-1797) was known as "The Town Destroyer," and "The Killer of Women and Children," among the Onadaga Indian People. Would you still respect him if you knew he was so prejudiced against the Native Americans that he once described them as "having nothing human except the shape" and as "a beast of prey?" Did he believe this country was founded upon Christian fundamentals? Washington is quoted as saying, "The United States is in no sense founded upon Christian doctrine."

By using the term Christianity, I am referring to all belief systems that base their practice upon the teachings of Jesus Christ. To be a true Christian, one must adhere to the principles of its founder. Jesus' teachings gave emphasis to statements such as "love one another as much as you love yourself," and "do unto others as you would have them do unto you," and "judge not so you will not be judged" and "there is no condemnation."

Washington's mistreatment of the Native Americans was anything but representative of Christian behavior. No matter what title we give ourselves, our actions speak louder than our words.

John Adams, the second President of the United States, had little use for Christianity when he said, "The divinity of Jesus is

71

made a convenient cover for absurdity. Nowhere in the Gospels do we find a precept for creeds, confessions, oaths, doctrines, and whole carloads of other foolish trumpery that we find in Christianity."

This is true. Many of the doctrines and creeds upheld by Christianity are man-made. I will explain this later.

The U.S. signed a Treaty of Peace and Friendship with Tripoli on November 4, 1796. It was signed again by Joel Barlow, the American consul general to the Barbary States at Algiers, on January 3, 1797. Barlow translated the text from its original Arabic language into English before it was ratified by President John Adams on June 10, 1797. Article 11 of the English version of the treaty reads:

> *As the government of the United States of America is not in any sense founded on the Christian religion as it has in itself no character of enmity against the laws, religion or tranquility of Musselmen [Muslims] and as the said States [America] have never entered into any war or act of hostility against any Mahometan nation, it is declared by the parties that no pretext arising from religious opinions shall ever produce an interruption of the harmony existing between the two countries.* [18]

Thomas Jefferson, the third President of the United States, and the principal author of the Declaration of Independence, "found not one redeeming feature in Orthodox Christianity" and added, "It does me no injury for my neighbor to say there are twenty gods or no God. It neither picks my pocket nor breaks my leg." Jefferson did not approve of religion having a voice in the government:

RIGHT TO RECOVER—*Yvonne Perry*

Believing with you that religion is a matter that lies solely between man and his God, that he owes account to none other for his faith or his worship, that the legislative powers of government reach actions only, and not opinions, I contemplate with sovereign reverence that act of the whole American people which declared that their legislature should make no law respecting an establishment of religion, or prohibiting the free exercise thereof, thus building a wall of separation between Church and State.

Jefferson called for limitation on the power of the federal government, and was an advocate for the separation of church and state. His own statement proves that he did not believe the country should be founded upon Christianity:

The day will come when the mystical generation of Jesus, by the Supreme Being as his Father, in the womb of a virgin, will be classified with the fable of the generation of Minerva in the brain of Jupiter. But we may hope that the dawn of reason and the freedom of thought in these United States will do away with this artificial scaffolding, and restore to us the primitive and genuine doctrines of this most venerated Reformer of human errors.

James Madison, fourth President of the United States, thought no better of the religion when he said:

During almost fifteen centuries the legal establishment known as Christianity has been on trial, and what have been the fruits, more or less, in all places? These are the fruits: pride, indolence, ignorance, and arrogance in the clergy. Ignorance, arrogance, and servility in the laity, and in both clergy and laity, superstition, bigotry, and persecution.

Abraham Lincoln, the 16th President of the United States,

was no doubt a religious man who is remembered as a Christian president; however, some say Lincoln was skeptical of Christianity. He is quoted as saying, "The Bible is not my Book and Christianity is not my religion. I could never give assent to the long complicated statements of Christian dogma." His views did not change during his political career. "My earlier views of the unsoundness of the Christian scheme of salvation and the human origin of the scriptures, have become clearer and stronger with advancing years and I see no reason for thinking I shall ever change them," said Lincoln.

After Lincoln's assassination, an American author and the editor of *Scribner's Monthly* named Dr. Josiah G. Holland wrote about Lincoln's religious views:

> "——He believed in God, and——believed himself to be under his control and guidance.——This unwavering faith in a Divine Providence began at his mother's knee, and ran like a thread of gold through all the experiences of his life. His constant sense of human duty was one of the forms by which his faith manifested itself. ——He recognized an immediate relation between God and himself, in all the actions and passions of his life. He was not professedly a Christian——that is, he subscribed to no creed——joined no organization of Christian disciples. He spoke little——of his religious belief and experiences; but that he had a deep religious life, sometimes imbued with superstition——."

Aside from former American presidents, other founding fathers of renown agree that Christianity has little merit when it comes to governing a nation of people. When Benjamin Franklin was asked about his religion, he said:

RIGHT TO RECOVER—*Yvonne Perry*

As to Jesus of Nazareth, I think the system of morals and his religion, as he left them to us, the best the world ever saw or is likely to see; but I apprehend it has received various corrupting changes, and I have, with the most of the present dissenters in England, some doubts to his divinity. ...I do not perceive that the Supreme takes it amiss, by distinguishing the unbelievers in his government of the world with any peculiar marks of his displeasure.

Deism is a seventeenth- and eighteenth-century religious philosophy and movement prominent in England and the United States. Deists normally reject supernatural events and divine revelation common to organized religion. Disregarding holy books and religions that affirm the existence of such things, deists support religious beliefs must be founded on human reason and observation of the natural world which reveals the existence of a supreme being. Deist Thomas Paine had a strong opinion about religion:

I do not believe in the creed professed by the Jewish Church, by the Roman Church, by the Greek Church, by the Turkish Church, by the Protestant Church, nor by any Church that I know of. My own mind is my own Church. ...Of all the tyrannies that affect mankind, tyranny in religion is the worst.

The First Amendment to the Constitution of the United States is part of the Bill of Rights which prevents legislation that establishes a national religion by Congress or that prefers or supports one religion over another. The First Amendment reads, "Congress shall make no law respecting an establishment of religion, or prohibiting the free exercise thereof." This part of the First Amendment is sometimes referred to as "the separation of church and state" which means that the state or national government should be kept separate from religious institutions.

Our founding fathers proposed the First Amendment and rejected Christianity as a ruling factor in government and political issues. After being ruled by a government which tried to synchronize the beliefs of the entire population, they were fed up with being told what to do and what to believe. They wanted religious freedom. The dream was short-lived. Soon after the early government of America was established, the same double-headed demon of politics and religion quickly rose to power. Many people who were healers (medical professionals), herbalists (pharmacologists), and midwives (obstetricians) were hunted down as witches and were tortured or burned at the stake in the northeastern U.S.–Salem, Massachusetts in particular.

The justification for killing witches was based upon assumptions made by those who were afraid of the healing power these individuals manifested. Rather than try to understand them, or their supernatural gifts, they judged these men and women as evil and condemned them to death.

Children are not inherently judgmental of others. Prejudice is a learned behavior that many carry on to adulthood. It's natural for adults to discredit and undermine things and people they do not understand. Rather than asking questions or researching origins, we judge harshly and reject others who believe differently than we do. If a behavior can be learned, it can be un-learned.

Even thinking about how common it was then to be killed for being "different" makes me shudder. I wish I could say things were different now and that we don't judge or banish those who have a different understanding of God, spiritual gifts, lifestyle preferences, or stem cell research, but, unfortunately, we do still take sides and throw stones at one another. For example, Codex

RIGHT TO RECOVER—*Yvonne Perry*

Alimentarius Commission was created in 1962 to regulate every aspect of how food and nutritional supplements are produced and sold to the consumer. The pharmaceutical industry has been working through Codex in the U.S. to pass laws that are friendly to their drug companies but hostile toward vitamins, minerals and supplements. Politicians and the U.S. government support Codex. Many occupations that utilize psychic or healing gifts and holistic (natural) or alternative therapies are thought to be inferior while medical doctors are one of the most respected vocations, and drug companies have people dependent upon them to provide services and products that were once considered "of the devil." We don't need the government making our medical decisions for us. As American citizens we have a right to work with our doctors to get the best possible healthcare available.

Our forefathers used religion to judge others without ever trying to understand something that was unfamiliar to them. I would have to say not much has changed to remove the bias against non-mainstream religions. Upon discovering a Wiccan coven in Oregon Township, Michigan, local residents freaked out and urged the town council and Representative John Stahl to "shut down the devil worshippers." This is a silly statement since Wiccans do not worship the devil—they don't even believe in one! Representative Stahl promised to "help get rid of" the coven while knowing that the law has recognized Wicca as a federally recognized religion since 1985. Its members have every right to practice their rituals as any other religion. While every religion has its quirky practices, it's not fair to stereotype and judge non-traditional religions. Earth-based religions still scare people. Some people believe that Pagans, Wiccans, and witches use animals in ritual sacrifice.

I know you are wondering what rabbit trail I'm going on now,

77

but, if you'll bear with me, I'll show you how so many people have come to believe and accept doctrine that is not based on truth—much like the belief that blastocyst stem cell research kills embryos.

Religious Tolerance?

I've done quite a bit of research on Paganism and other Earth-based religions and happen to know that Wiccans are not apt to practice animal sacrifice. In fact many of them are vegans who support animal rights. However, there are many Christians who believe every word of the Bible—a book that contains multiple references to animal sacrifice. The Old Testament of the Bible supported the ritual of animal sacrifice to Jehovah or Yahweh, the God of the Jews. It stands to reason that anyone who believes that the Bible is the infallible word of God also believes animal sacrifice is an acceptable form of worship—although not needed in New Testament times since Jesus is considered a human sacrifice. *Did I say human sacrifice?* Religions are built on principles such as these, and we accept the beliefs as "normal." Think about how outlandish and disempowering martyrdom really is.

So, why is it a big deal if someone kills an animal as part of a religious practice? From what I've studied about religions that use animal sacrifice in ritual, the meat is eaten rather than wasted, and the spirit of the animal is respectfully asked to give up its life for the purpose of helping a human recover or for good fortune in battle or other human pursuits. That's better treatment than most animals get when facing the slaughter house, wouldn't you agree?

More than 95 percent of Americans are meat eaters. This means most of us don't have a problem with an animal being killed for a human to have dinner. These animals are not treated humanely; the environment in which they are raised is atrocious! The poultry and cattle industries are financially assisted by the government to maximize profits. That means they are encouraged to put growth hormones, vaccines, and preservative chemicals into the meat.

Just think of all the people who eat turkey on Thanksgiving Day. We were thankful for the sacrifice of life! And, those birds weren't even sacrificed to a deity…or were they? Yes, they were sacrificed to the gods of greed and gluttony. Which one of us is not guilty? When it comes to animal sacrifice, let a vegan cast the first stone.

Okay, everyone has a right to believe however they choose, so let's get back on the topic at hand.

Due to interpretation of the First Amendment, the separation of church and state has been a topic of political debate throughout American history. Some people say that the language does not prohibit the government's entry into religious issues in order to achieve the purposes of the Free Exercise Clause of the First Amendment. Obviously, the government has no right of jurisdiction on sacred issues or to aid any particular religion or its philosophies. Nevertheless, the government is already involved in the religious and political interests surrounding blastocyst stem cell research. A few religious radical right-wing members and one man have used their religious persuasion to prevent federal funding of IV-B research. This is the same man who, without Congressional approval or guidance, and without judicial review, succeeded in opening the checkbooks of five federal departments to religious organizations. After failing to persuade Congress to change the law, President Bush rewrote regulations that annually released multi-billions of federal taxpayer dollars to religious groups to supplement or support their social services programs with no Congressional oversight. This is clearly a violation of the Establishment Clause of the First Amendment.

And, thanks to a Supreme Court ruling in a 1968 court case, *Flast v Cohen*, U.S. taxpayers do not have a right to sue in an attempt to stop the spending of money that violates our Constitution. On February 28, 2007, the Supreme Court heard arguments in *Hein v Freedom from Religion Foundation*. This case threatens to make the federal government completely immune from challenges when it spends money to support religion. The Bush-created Office of Faith-Based and Community Initiatives gives money directly to a religious school or organization.

There can be no religious freedom whenever religion controls the masses through the government. Yet, this is exactly what has occurred in the U.S. Each time a law is passed giving government jurisdiction over what happens in a person's home, marriage, healthcare or religion, we lose another personal right that was assured to us in the founding documents of our country.

Time and time again, religious groups have violated our Constitutional right to keep church and state separate. The neoconservative and fundamentalists' unfounded opinion about blastocyst stem cell research is hindering the physical and financial health of our nation. Yes, I do mean financial health. Not only will people spend less on treating symptoms, but the jobs, companies, and income that stand to be created by stem cell technology will benefit our nation both physically and financially.

Most of my readers are not in the right-wing groups that oppose the research. You are curious to know more about it in order to form your own opinion. The people this book will not reach are the religious right-wingers who have given total allegiance to their church, pastor, denomination, or Bible and allow political and religious leaders to rule their thinking. These are people who are not willing to think for themselves or who are afraid to break away from family traditions and fear-based belief systems that have been handed down to them. Never stopping to ask why their theology doesn't fit their experience, they accept dogma that doesn't make sense. They do not realize such things are being used to control them. People continue to adhere to standards of practice and outdated thinking even when it doesn't work for them. I was one of them. I understand where they are coming from.

Being raised in a conservative Baptist church, my religious training started when I was two weeks old and my parents dedicated me to God. As I grew up, I never questioned my family's strict, yet inconsistent, hypocritical moral code until I became a teenager. Even then, I never got into any serious trouble as I left home at seventeen to marry. My first husband and I raised our children in an independent, severely fundamental, Baptist Church where everything was taboo. Sin was spelled "f-u-n" so, if there was fun to be had, we couldn't join in. When my marriage ended 22 years later, I began to question everything I had ever been taught and found that many of my religious beliefs no longer served me. Still praying for hours each day, religion and doctrine could not help me as I plummeted into depression and despair. In fact, those who had been my friends in the church scolded me for not having enough faith to prevent my divorce. So much for Christians being known for their love; judgment was all I received in the darkest hour of my soul. I had broken the rules of my religion, and my religion no longer accepted me.

That was a turning point in my life. I realized that much of what I had been taught in a religious setting was damaging to my emotions. Some fundamentalists love a martyr to the point that they teach codependency, female subservience, and total allegiance to their leaders. I had been taught that a wife should submit to the rule of her husband, to never question God or her pastor, and that all the circumstances in my life were not my fault—it was simply God's will for me to suffer. I was disempowered to believe that I was not responsible for my miserable life, so I kept waiting for God to bail me out or change my situation.

All throughout my religious years, I felt like a misfit because inwardly I didn't really agree with the doctrine of my religion. I often tried to balk the system when certain "rules" were being enforced within the congregation. This caused the leaders to see me as a threat to their power. I was often rejected or asked to leave a fellowship for voicing an opinion that questioned authority of the leadership or the validity of the church's rules and regulations. Thinking for yourself weakens the stronghold another person has upon you.

I ended my relationship with religious establishments in 2001 and sought my own path to find my connection that already existed with my Creator. That connection was not based on rules or tradition. As I moved away from the system of religion, and put aside the "to-do" list of the Church, I began to trust my intuition and heed the inner voice I had been ignoring for years. I began to take personal responsibility for my choices, and I regained my power as I exercised free will rather than allowing people to walk all over me. I researched and studied all types of religion and found both truth and myths in each one. I found that the Bible has been altered many times to serve the agendas of politicians and leaders of the early Church and Roman government.

Those who have done little or no research on stem cells adhere to the belief that an IV-B is an embryo. Why? Because someone they look to for leadership has told them it is true. Whether it pertains to IV-B research or your religious dogma, do you know why you believe what you do? Are your beliefs your own? Do you know the origins of your religion? If you are reading this book, you must be a truth seeker who is open minded enough to bear with me as I continue to challenge your beliefs. Let's look more closely at how Christianity evolved to its modern day system of beliefs.

How Did Christianity Get Started?

There are three main branches of modern Christianity: Protestantism (meaning to protest) initiated by Martin Luther's 95 Theses and rooted in the Protestant Reformation adhering to the Scriptures as the authority for one's life; Catholicism adhering to the Christian Nicene Creed in 325 A.D. while maintaining authority over the scriptures; and Eastern Orthodoxy adhering to church traditions descending from the Eastern Roman Empire or Byzantium.

When the Old Religion of the Pagan culture was taken over by Christianity, Pagans kept some of their traditions hidden within the practice of the dominant religion. The Celtic cross is an important symbol to both faiths. Based on older Pagan designs, it represents the earth and the four elements: air, fire, water, and earth. When forced to trace it on their chests, Pagans consciously affirmed it as a symbol of their own faith rather than a symbol of the Church. The Celts continued to honor their gods and goddesses by disguising them as Catholic saints. The Pagan goddess Bride became known as St. Brigid. In the centre of the town of Carnac in Brittany, France, is a Catholic church dedicated to Saint Cornely—the patron saint of horned beasts. This is actually Cernunnos, the old Pagan god of the hunt cleaned up, de-horned, dressed up, and canonized. When Christian priests realized their heavy approach was not working to rid the world of the Old Religion, they began quietly creating Catholic versions of the old gods. Even the Virgin Mother Mary is a representation of the Goddess herself.

I'm not here to espouse one religion or condemn another. Any world history or religion class will clearly show that modern-day Western Christianity is certainly not based on the true teachings of the mystical prophet and teacher Jesus Christ of Nazareth and that the Bible is not the infallible word of God many people think it is. Old Testament stories were passed down orally in Hebrew from the time of Abraham to Jesus. The way vowels and consonants are pronounced give Hebrew words their meaning. If one vowel is pronounced incorrectly, the word could mean something entirely different. From oral to written, there could be even more margin for error. Originally the New Testament was written in Aramaic except for the Greek writings of Paul.

As Jews spread throughout the Roman Empire, they began to lose their native language, the 39 books of the Hebrew Old Testament and the Apocrypha (Judith, Tobit, Baruch, Ecclesiasticus, the Wisdom of Solomon, First and Second Maccabees, Esdras, Esther, Daniel, and the Prayer of Manasseh) were translated into the Greek language. The Septuagint (Latin for seventy) is named after the seventy Jewish scholars who were commissioned between 300-200 B.C. to translate these Jewish Scriptures into a language that could be read by early non-Hebrew Christians during the first few centuries A.D. Protestant Christians or Orthodox Jews do not consider the Apocryphal books as part of the Bible.

Christianity has gone through many transformations over the

years, and the religion people in the U.S. practice today is not at all like it was in the beginning. True Christianity has Jesus Christ as its focal point, not rules and regulation; not dogma or doctrine. Christianity began with the gentle, non-violent teachings of Jesus Christ for whom the religion is named. Jesus' teachings were in alignment with Buddhist, Tibetan, and Eastern thought that did not adhere to religious or political authority but rather supported an individualistic, anti-materialist, non-political lifestyle. Jews who followed the teachings of Christ were just beginning to adapt the principles into their culture when non-Jews (Greek and Roman) began to adopt the religion as their own. The Gospels, which give account of the life of Christ, were written at least 30 to 70 years after the death of Jesus. Paul of Tarsus is one of the earliest founders of the Greek/Roman version of Christianity who penned parts of the New Testament. Paul's writings, which espouse subjection of women and paying homage to pastors and church leaders, actually oppose the early teachings of Jesus.

The Nicene Creed

The Old Religion (Pantheism) was tolerant of diverse religious practices. When Christianity became the state religion of Rome, it merged with the older polytheistic and mythological belief systems. However, when the emperor Constantine took the throne in 302 A.D. he did not like the hodge-podge and various forms of Christianity because they lacked a uniform doctrine. Constantine wanted complete authority over his kingdom, and he set out to change things. He called together the Christian bishops at Nicæa and hashed out a new doctrine that came to be known as the Nicene Creed, which is commonly recited by Eastern Orthodox, Roman Catholics, Anglicans, Lutherans, Calvinists, and many other

Christian groups. I place the text here so you may see the wording and framework for the new doctrine.

We believe in one God, the Father, the Almighty, maker of heaven and earth, of all that is, seen and unseen. We believe in one Lord, Jesus Christ, the only son of God, eternally begotten of the Father, God from God, Light from Light, true God from true God, begotten, not made, of one being with the Father. Through him all things were made. For us and for our salvation he came down from heaven: by the power of the Holy Spirit he became incarnate from the Virgin Mary, and was made man. For our sake he was crucified under Pontius Pilate; he suffered death and was buried. On the third day he rose again in accordance with the Scriptures; he ascended into heaven and is seated at the right hand of the Father. He will come again in glory to judge the living and the dead, and his kingdom will have no end. We believe in the Holy Spirit, the Lord, the giver of life, who proceeds from the Father [and the Son]. With the Father and the Son he is worshipped and glorified. He has spoken through the Prophets. We believe in one holy catholic and apostolic Church. We acknowledge one baptism for the forgiveness of sins. We look for the resurrection of the dead, and the life of the world to come. AMEN.

The Nicene Council also compiled the New Testament, which included Judaic works such as the letters of Jude and John, and excerpts from Paul's letters that were misaligned with the peaceful teachings of Jesus Christ. The New Testament excluded the Gospel of Philip because it exposed dishonest leadership and supported reincarnation. Many people today believe the Bible is the inspired, infallible Word of God, but, as you can see here, it is a text that has been compiled by political rulers and altered many times throughout its course.

RIGHT TO RECOVER—*Yvonne Perry*

The compassionate and tender principles contained in the early history of true Christianity started to fade as the Orthodox Church of Rome continued to develop a doctrine that would enable political rulers to enslave citizens and force the congregation to materially support pastors and obey them without question. Of course, this new view of Christianity was not liked by humble Christians of that day. Arius was a major opponent of the new doctrine, which taught that humans are sinners as a result of the fall of Adam and Eve. This doctrine of "original sin" has been carried over to fundamentalist religions today that teach people that they are destined to hell if they do not submit to certain beliefs and practices. Special status was given to church leaders. These pastors, bishops, and church elders were said to be the only ones who could forgive sin and save people from hell. They required people to do service for the church, give a tithe to support the pastors, and even take up arms against the enemies of the church. Arius was one such historical enemy. A decree was issued and enforced stating that anyone who read or followed Arius' teachings would be killed.

Another ruling of this new religion declared the human body sinful and prohibited a couple to have sexual relations without permission from the Church. This is where belief in the virgin birth (that Mary the mother of Jesus conceived and gave birth without losing her virginity) was manufactured. Children who were conceived and born without the Church's permission were not eligible for Baptism or forgiveness of sins—of course, unless the parents paid penance or gave money to the bishop. This is also when the belief began that Jesus is the only son of God. And, that really doesn't make sense to me. The peace-loving Jesus himself stated that we are all sons and daughters of God; equal to Him— joint heirs with full rights and responsibilities as co-creators of our lives and our circumstances. The illusion of separateness from

God or our Creative Source is strange. It is in the Creator that we all live and have our being.

The idea of humans being depraved sinners has placed leaders of certain religious sects in a lofty place of superiority. Believing that one is exclusive and special to God for having believed the mandates of a certain religious doctrine isolates people from others who believe differently. All of us are organs, vessels, tissues, limbs, appendages, and body parts that make up the "many members" the Bible refers to as the "body and bride of Christ." This "oneness" is a common principle in many Eastern religions.

European cultures from 400 A.D. and through the Renaissance adopted, and further altered, Christianity to fit their diverse multicultural societies. It is plain to see that what started out as Christianity is nothing like what it is today. Unfortunately, some aggressive, fundamental, evangelical Christians still spread hate and animosity against people who worship any deity other than Jesus Christ, or who practice any lifestyle unlike their own. All the while, the teachings they think belong to Jesus actually belong to a political and religious system that breeds hate and fear. If you are willing to see Christianity in a new light, I suggest you read *Why Christianity Must Change or Die* by Bishop John Shelby Spong or *Misquoting Jesus* by Bart Erhman. Be warned that these books challenge the Apostle's Creed and many other spiritual beliefs passed down through history.

Some people say God never changes. However, I find contradiction with the god of the Bible who condemns murder in the "Thou Shalt Not" list of rules and goes into battle to help the Israelites slay thousands of people in another passage of text. This is because our beloved deities are made in the likeness of man, and we have forgotten our likeness to the Creator. We have given divine primordial energy, or creative life force, both negative and positive personality traits and characteristics in order to worship it. And, we use our gods to do battle and force our opinions on one another—even to influence our government to prohibit federal funding for a life-saving research. Truly, our connection with the Divine is found within our spirit—not within an organization, creed, or person.

An undifferentiated blastocyst stem cell can become any type of cell under ideal conditions. Therefore, I compare these cells to the original "nothingness" that contains the potential for any and everything that can be, or has been, created. For a moment, I want you to lay aside your preconceived ideas about whom or what God is and think of our Creator as the original stem cell or immortal energy. This energy has differentiated into the multi-faceted body of humanity and even includes planets, stars, and universes. Perhaps God is the figurative Adam (masculine side of the Creator) and we are Eve, the Goddess or feminine energy bifurcated from a Source that contains both male and female energies. Male and female are two sides of the same coin. Unlike the teachings of male-dominant religions, masculine and feminine energies are equal. One cannot exist without the other. Just as God/Goddess cannot be destroyed, neither can life. Both are energy, which can only be changed from one thing to another.

No one can explain God, not religion, not even science; nevertheless, I hope you enjoyed my Metaphysics 101 class.

I imagine most of my readers are compassionate people who have a love for their Creator and fellow humans. I applaud you for stepping out of the mold and being true to yourself. Many of you are Christians who would love to see the original teachings and examples set by Jesus Christ enacted in daily life, government, and church-related activities. Christ's teachings are not found on tablets of stone or within the paper pages of any text. The book of the Law is written on our hearts and must be accessed internally. Some people worship the Bible instead of following their internal guidance. Our divine self would not lead us to become war-loving, judgmental people. Those are the ones who disgrace other believers by calling themselves Christians.

Religion certainly has its place, and I hate to think of where our society would be without the moral guidance of good people. Religion gives us a feeling of community and belonging and may be very important to those who are displaced from their biological families. Religion serves some people in finding their identity with like-minded others. Religion can help some reconnect with their Creator, but beware of tenets which dictate that humans are sinful beings separate from God. No one should tell another person they are a sinner or going to hell if they do not conform to a certain standard—that's judgment and condemnation. Jesus taught love and acceptance even for an adulterous woman shunned by society. Beware of any teachings or organization that says you must behave a certain way or believe a particular doctrine in order to be accepted by God or allowed into the Divine kingdom. The greatest gift of all is that of free will. Many religions attempt to take that away from its followers.

When you are able to step back from your belief system and assess its origins, you may find that you really don't "own" your truth. You simply believe what someone else told you. The generations who passed down their traditions and beliefs to you have not traced those traditions and beliefs back to their roots. I can't over emphasize how dangerous it is to give away your free will and personal power to any religious or political leader.

RIGHT TO RECOVER—*Yvonne Perry*

Is there Hope for the Religious Crowd?

There is a huge difference between religion and spirituality. Our spirituality has to do with our inward connection with the Divine; religion has to do with outward rules and regulations. Everyone is a spiritual being, but not everyone claims to be religious.

I was a religious addict for many years! Ask my children. I was locked away in a prayer room for hours each day as they were growing up. Homework, dinner, band practice, and anything else they needed would have to wait until I finished wearing God out with my supplication. I was at church at least five times a week, either for praise band rehearsal, prayer meeting, Bible study, or worship services. I also participated in inner-city evangelism and hosted prayer and praise groups in my home. I looked down upon anyone who was not as "good" as me. It seemed normal at the time, but as I look back at those fanatical times, I realize I was not really "present" in my home, marriage, or family. I'm sure it had a detrimental effect upon my kids, but somehow they have managed to forgive me.

There is not a single religion I can call my own. Instead, I honor all paths and allow others to believe whatever they want to as long as it doesn't harm me or those I love. I draw the line at keeping silent when another person's religion prevents funding for research that has a high potential for helping heal my quadriplegic friends and my family members who have diabetes and other illnesses. If I can change, anyone can.

In fact, the eyes of some other "dyed-in-the-wool" religious folks are beginning to open. I interviewed Jim Palmer as a guest on my podcast *Writers in the Sky*. His book *Divine Nobodies* is about shedding religion to find God. Once the evangelistic pastor of a mega-church, Jim's faithful followers rejected him when his marriage ended in divorce. Through people who did not fit the

Christian mold, Jim found his true connection with Christ and dropped the façade of "doing" church.

Reverend Mel White terminated his long-term career as the ghostwriter for religious right leaders Pat Robertson and Jerry Falwell. White is now a member of Defcon (Defending the Constitution of America) and is confronting the hate-filled, religion-based, homophobic, racist scheme against fellow Americans. He is the author of *Religion Gone Bad,* which exposes the true agenda of these fundamental extremists. DefCon is an online grassroots movement combating the growing power of the religious right. Their concern is for the separation of church and state, individual freedom, scientific progress, pluralism, and tolerance while respecting people of faith and their right to express their beliefs.

I sincerely believe that Dan Bloodworth's religious affiliation and Biblical support for research on blastocyst stem cells is a valuable tool for educating right-wing conservatives who adamantly oppose stem cell research.

For 65 years Former President Jimmy Carter was a member of the Southern Baptist denomination—the nation's largest Protestant denomination. In 2000, he and his wife disassociated from the church due to its "increasingly rigid creed" that prohibits women from being pastors and tells wives to be submissive to their husbands.

I've given five instances where people are getting real with themselves and letting go of the crutches of religion to become who they are destined to be, or, should I say, who they were all along—children of the Divine; sparks from the flame of the Creator.

I hope you will not be offended at my opposition to Westernized Christianity. It is the system I'm against, not the peace-loving, non-prejudiced, global citizens who happen to call themselves by a term that is extremely misrepresentative of its founder. My rebuttal is not intended to criticize anyone but to get us all thinking about what is going on in the name of religion.

Now, let's look at the political side of the opposition to blastocyst stem cell research.

Chapter Five

REBUTTAL OF PRESIDENT
BUSH'S STATEMENT

George W. Bush's vetoing H.R. 810 was an insult to millions of suffering people, and he didn't stop a single "murder" in the process! Just as many blastocysts are being thrown in the trash as were before. He refuses to support H.R. 3 (also known as S-5 The Stem Cell Research Enhancement Act) or other bills that favor research on blastocyst stem cells. More than seventy percent of the people in America approve of blastocyst stem cell research, yet the wishes of the majority are not being carried out by those we have elected to represent us.

The Bush Administration questions the morality of research that destroys human embryos, yet according to our Constitution it is neither the government's business nor right to legislate morality. However, under the rule of our present government there is very little separation of Church and State.

In an address to the nation on stem cell research, President Bush said:

> *I also believe human life is a sacred gift from our Creator. I worry about a culture that devalues life, and believe as your President*

RIGHT TO RECOVER—*Yvonne Perry*

I have an important obligation to foster and encourage respect for life in America and throughout the world. And while we're all hopeful about the potential of this research, no one can be certain that the science will live up to the hope it has generated.[19]

Everyone, not just our leaders, has an obligation to respect life globally. I agree that human life is a sacred gift from our Creator. All life is sacred. However, an IVF-derived blastocyst is a cluster of living but undifferentiated cells, and not an entire organism—much less a human being. These spheres of cells are only a few days old and were created in a laboratory. They are not even visible to the naked eye. They do not have body parts, nerve or blood cells; they have yet to become anything! They are undefined, which means that under certain conditions they could become tissue, cells, organs, blood vessels, or, if unhindered in the natural environment of the womb, they could develop into a human being. However, at the point in which these cells are taken for research, they have not taken the form of a human being.

From the Johns Hopkins Medicine essay co-written by professors Faden and Gearhart:

> *We believe that most Americans have different moral values from the president's. While we recognize and respect embryos as early forms of human life, we do not believe that embryos in a dish have the same moral status as children and adults. We believe that the obligation to relieve human suffering binds us all and justifies the instrumental use of early embryonic life. And we believe that it is possible to draw morally relevant lines and to enforce them as a matter of national policy.*[20]

In their email to me, Joe and Nina Brown of Bellaire, Texas make a good point about how blastocyst stem cells are a gift from God.

95

RIGHT TO RECOVER—*Yvonne Perry*

As the centuries have gone by, God has revealed more and more of His wonders to us as we have become ready to receive them. He has given us the ability, coupled with the responsibility, to recognize His gifts as He presents them......Throughout the history of mankind God has continued to reveal ever-increasing life-enhancing knowledge, from herbs to the microscope, surgery, pharmaceuticals and nuclear medicine. We believe that God has chosen to reveal this 14-day window of opportunity before the cells begin to differentiate, as His gift to sustain and prolong life and relieve human suffering. After which, He has given us the gift of creation of life. For both gifts, we thank God.

In July 2006, Presidential Press Secretary Tony Snow said that George W. Bush had to veto increased federal funding for blastocystic stem cell research because the president is against murder. I'm not sure I believe that. After all, he is adamant about sending in more troops to be killed in Iraq.

Since most of the blastocyst stem cell lines approved by Mr. Bush are not suitable to the development of human therapies, researchers and doctors must have a fresh supply for transplantation. Dr. Curt Freed (University of Colorado Health Sciences Center) uses blastocyst stem cells to make dopamine cells suitable for the brains of Parkinson's patients and to create insulin cells needed to treat diabetes. He has no other source to pull from. Doctors like these should never be equated to murderers. They don't kill; they heal!

"Tens of thousands of frozen embryos are thrown away every year," said Dr. Freed. "It has nothing to do with murder. It has to do with wasting a precious resource. If converting frozen embryos to embryonic stem cells is murder, what is throwing them in the trash?"[21]

RIGHT TO RECOVER—*Yvonne Perry*

Thou Shalt Not Kill. Oh, Really?

Murder in the name of religion and politics is not new. The Crusades, the Spanish Inquisition, and most political events during the Dark Ages were initiated by religious authorities who wanted to control the masses. What better way to do this than by regulating the beliefs of an entire nation through fear of death or persecution? Are we any wiser and more humane in the 21st century? Greed, control, and killing in the name of religion still exist. While fundamental, dogmatic religions in America do not blatantly kill people who believe differently than them, they do excommunicate anyone who challenges their authority or belief system. Or at least that was my experience. These fundamentalist neoconservative religious leaders support war efforts that kill innocent people, but they will be the first to tell you that abortion for any reason is murder. Pope Benedict XVI, formerly known as Cardinal Joseph Ratzinger, ordered U.S. bishops to deny communion to members of their congregation who openly support abortion rights because they are guilty of a "grave sin." What a childish act to reject and punish someone for having beliefs that differ from the "authority" of the Church.

Our President and most of his right-wing followers agree that war (murder) is allowable for the greater good of all. I am concerned about the society we live in that devalues life by supporting war the way ours does. Perhaps it's not our society who devalues life, but rather a minority of Senators and our President. As of January 2007, the U.S. government is spending $8 billion a month to fund the war in Iraq but refuses to spend millions to preserve or enhance life or to find cures for debilitating conditions and diseases. After President Bush's address in January 2007, Associated Press-Ipsos telephone survey of 1,002 adults showed that seventy percent of the American people are opposed to his suggestion of sending an additional 21,500 troops to Iraq.

The Lancet is a highly respected British medical journal, which estimated in December 2006 that 650,000 Iraqis have died as a result of the war that started in 2003. That's almost twice the estimated 300,000 people killed by Saddam Hussein during his 23 years of brutal rule. More American soldiers have died in the Iraq war (3,008 and counting) than were killed in the 9-11 attacks in New York, Washington, and Pennsylvania (2,794). A growing number of conservatives openly challenging the administration's war tactics have agreed that a full military victory to establish democracy in Iraq is not possible. Senator John McCain said American troops in Iraq were "fighting and dying for a failed policy."

Pro-Life and Anti-Stem Cell Research?

Why are pro-war people upset about frozen cells being used for research? It doesn't make sense for anyone to say they are pro-life and be in favor of war at the same time. It seems contradictory to say that the allocation of a blastocyst to science is evil, while the killing of adults is acceptable.

I suppose the sixth of the Ten Commandments has a "kick out" clause. Certainly in our culture "thou shall not kill" is a rule that may be bent for political purposes or self-defense. It's easy to see where the mentality of blood-shed religion came from. Holy wars (war is anything *but* holy) still exist between countries that have been feuding for generations with other nations who disagree with their doctrine or politics. According to the Bible, God's prophet, Elijah, killed 400 prophets of Baal in a contest of wills, which engaged a supernatural show of power between Elijah's God and Baal, the god worshipped by Jezebel and her cohorts. In other words, if you don't agree with us, we will kill you; and our God not only approves of it, He will help us kill you! Thankfully, my Jewish friends are not so hotheaded!

Frank Cocozzelli with the Institute for Progressive Christianity says:

> *If President Bush was truly pro-life, why did he—(and other research opponents) take hundreds of thousands of dollars in campaign contributions from tobacco special interest groups? Consider this: tobacco has the potential to end lives; but embryonic stem cell and somatic cell nuclear transfer research have the potential to save lives.*[22]

According to C. Everett Koop, Republican, former Surgeon General of the United States, tobacco causes spontaneous abortion, premature birth, and low birth weight. As many as 100,000 newborn babies die before birth due to tobacco use during pregnancy. New data also show that permanent fetal brain damage and disabilities are caused by tobacco, including problems such as attention deficit hyperactivity disorder.

Both Democrats and Republicans take campaign contributions from the tobacco industry. However, 80% of the $6,033,226 in funds donated by tobacco companies went to Republican Party committees and only 20% went to Democrat Party committees in the 2001-2002 election. George Bush has been in association with the tobacco industry and its lobbyists since he was the Governor of Texas. As president, G.W. Bush gives "breaks" to the tobacco industry by lessening the severity of fines in class-action law suits against them.

President George W. Bush vetoed the Stem Cell Research Enhancement Act on what he claimed were "pro-life" grounds. But how can an elected official call himself pro-life, pro-child, pro-family while supporting an industry that is responsible for literally millions of deaths? How could he allow his campaign to be funded by the makers of tobacco that contains a dangerous drug that causes addiction in children?

What is Death?

We have assigned value to some things/people as good and others as bad. We are programmed to believe that death is a bad or tragic thing. Even if a death occurs, it can be considered a good thing because death is simply another side of life. It is the ending of one phase and the beginning of another. A soul is immortal. Our consciousness or soul essence does not end when we stop breathing or lose brain function.

In studying string theory, scientists are discovering that many dimensions exist simultaneously. We are multi-dimensional spirits having a human experience. Haven't you ever had a dream that was so real it was like you were really there? You probably were visiting other dimensions by astral travel. When a person dies, his spirit simply selects a new dimension in which to express itself without a human body. Whatever happens to the body is of no concern to the soul who has departed from it. It may very well be the same with a fetus that dies before reaching full term. Whatever happens to the "host" or fetal flesh does not bring any grief to the immortal soul. The soul that was intending to come in through that vehicle will simply move on and find another opportunity to incarnate.

Is murder wrong? Most Americans would say "yes." Those in tribal countries where savage warfare is a matter of survival would not think murder is wrong. Suicide bombers actually think they have done God and the world a favor by killing those who disagree with their religious or political opinions. So, when we

talk of abortion and blastocystic stem cell research, does right or
wrong really need to be a deciding factor? The endless political and
religious posturing on these issues is a waste of time. The imagery
of the potential life in an IV-B is damaging to the real lives of real
people hoping for cures. Shouldn't we agree to work together to
do whatever helps the most people live the best lives possible?
Wouldn't that be more in line with the teachings of Jesus Christ
who healed everyone he possibly could?

In *Religion and Science, New York Times Magazine*, November 9,
1930, Albert Einstein is quoted as saying, "A man's ethical behavior
should be based effectually on sympathy, education, and social ties
and needs; no religious basis is necessary. Man would indeed be in
a poor way if he had to be restrained by fear of punishment and
hope of reward after death."[23]

I've concluded that there is really no way to distinguish right
from wrong or define good and bad for the entire planet because
our definition of what is moral and what is unacceptable varies
from culture to culture and from person to person. Even those who
base their ethical guidelines upon the Bible have to deal with the
inconsistency of the text and the knowledge that the book has been
altered through the ages. Even then, our personal interpretation of
the text will vary. It appears to me that we each need to find our
own truth within ourselves and live by that.

Let's continue with my rebuttal to Bush's statement on policy
regarding blastocyst stem cell research. This speech was given in
Crawford, Texas in August 2001:[24]

*My administration must decide whether to allow federal
funds, your tax dollars, to be used for scientific research on stem cells
derived from human embryos. A large number of these embryos
already exist. They are the product of a process called in-vitro*

fertilization, which helps so many couples conceive children. When doctors match sperm and egg to create life outside the womb, they usually produce more embryos than are planted in the mother. Once a couple successfully has children, or if they are unsuccessful, the additional embryos remain frozen in laboratories.

Some will not survive during long storage; others are destroyed. A number have been donated to science and used to create privately funded stem cell lines. And a few have been implanted in an adoptive mother and born, and are today healthy children.

Bush is not giving credit to the female womb required in order for an embryo to exist. He is saying that a lab-created clump of cells is a human being. Continuing to propagate this misunderstanding only strengthens the belief in something that is scientifically impossible at this point in history. He continues:

Based on preliminary work that has been privately funded, scientists believe further research using stem cells offers great promise that could help improve the lives of those who suffer from many terrible diseases -- from Juvenile diabetes to Alzheimer's, from Parkinson's to spinal cord injuries. And while scientists admit they are not yet certain, they believe stem cells derived from embryos have unique potential.

Scientists further believe that rapid progress in this research will come only with federal funds. Federal dollars help attract the best and brightest scientists. They ensure new discoveries are widely shared at the largest number of research facilities and that the research is directed toward the greatest public good.

The United States has a long and proud record of leading the world toward advances in science and medicine that improve

RIGHT TO RECOVER—*Yvonne Perry*

human life. And the United States has a long and proud record of upholding the highest standards of ethics as we expand the limits of science and knowledge. Research on embryonic stem cells raises profound ethical questions, because extracting the stem cell destroys the embryo, and thus destroys its potential for life. Like a snowflake, each of these embryos is unique, with the unique genetic potential of an individual human being.

As I thought through this issue, I kept returning to two fundamental questions: First, are these frozen embryos human life, and therefore, something precious to be protected? And second, if they're going to be destroyed anyway, shouldn't they be used for a greater good, for research that has the potential to save and improve other lives?

I've asked those questions and others of scientists, scholars, bioethicists, religious leaders, doctors, researchers, members of Congress, my Cabinet, and my friends. I have read heartfelt letters from many Americans. I have given this issue a great deal of thought, prayer and considerable reflection. And I have found widespread disagreement.

On the first issue, are these embryos human life -- well, one researcher told me he believes this five-day-old cluster of cells is not an embryo, not yet an individual, but a pre-embryo. He argued that it has the potential for life, but it is not a life because it cannot develop on its own.

And, why does the President need further proof than that? Why does he continue to wage war on the millions of citizens who might benefit from blastocyst stem cell research? I cannot understand why a clump of cells is more important to him than a living, tax-paying human being.

RIGHT TO RECOVER—*Yvonne Perry*

An ethicist dismissed that as a callous attempt at rationalization. Make no mistake, he told me, that cluster of cells is the same way you and I, and all the rest of us, started our lives. One goes with a heavy heart if we use these, he said, because we are dealing with the seeds of the next generation.

Ejaculate material and menstrual blood also contain sperm and eggs that have the potential to become a human being, so shouldn't they be considered nascent life as well? Do we need a law about the proper use of such material? Oh, but the sperm and the egg have to be united/fertilized before they can become an embryo, they might argue. And I remind everyone that a fertilized egg has to be implanted in a woman's uterus before it can become an embryo or a human life. There is no way a clump of cells can become a human being in a Petri dish, no matter what chemical cocktail (even amniotic fluid) is used to coax it.

And to the other crucial question, if these are going to be destroyed anyway, why not use them for good purpose -- I also found different answers. Many argue these embryos are byproducts of a process that helps create life, and we should allow couples to donate them to science so they can be used for good purpose instead of wasting their potential. Others will argue there's no such thing as excess life, and the fact that a living being is going to die does not justify experimenting on it or exploiting it as a natural resource.

A living being? A plant is a living being. A rat is a living being. We do research on rats. A soldier is a living being not a natural resource to be wasted on a war that cannot be won.

Leading scientists tell me research on these 60 lines have great promise that could lead to breakthrough therapies and cures. This allows us to explore the promise and potential of stem cell research without crossing a fundamental moral line, by providing taxpayer funding that would sanction or encourage further destruction of human embryos that have at least the potential for life.

The cell lines that were supposed to have such great promise have been found to be unusable for research purposes because they were developed using animal feeder layers of cells. Being created in such a manner poses a risk of contamination with mouse viruses or proteins making these cell lines clinically unviable for human research or for treating diseases in humans.

Johns Hopkins professors Ruth Faden and John Gearhart explain:

The embryonic stem cell lines the president approved for federal funding three years ago, all of which were derived before August 2001, are clearly inadequate to advance stem cell science, let alone to take that science from the bench to the bedside. There are too few of them, no more than 21. All of the approved stem cell lines were prepared using mouse cells and thus pose a risk of contaminating human subjects with mouse viruses. This is a needless risk; since 2001 we have developed techniques for establishing embryonic stem cell lines without using mouse cells. Even if the approved lines were safe for use in humans, many patients who would be appropriate and willing participants in the first human trials would have difficulty receiving grafts based on these lines because of problems of genetic matching. There are just too few lines to even begin to accommodate the genetic diversity in our population. [25]

President Bush's statement continues:

I also believe that great scientific progress can be made through aggressive federal funding of research on umbilical cord placenta, *adult and animal stem cells which do not involve the same moral dilemma. This year, your government will spend $250 million on this important research.*

While I advocate we use all types of stem cells and provide federal funding for each, we know that adult stem cells do not have the same plasticity as younger stem cells. Stem cells from umbilical cord and placenta have already started differentiating into specific types of cells, organs, tissues, and vessels and, therefore, do not have the same capacity as IV-B stem cells. Blastocysts are not whole organisms having distinct or complete characteristics. They are not people, and they are not body parts, they are living cells! Cellular life requires nourishment and energy to sustain itself whether they are skin cells or liver cells. We have shown earlier that IV-B stem cells are not human embryos because they do not have blood in them, they do not have nerve or circulatory systems or other organs, and they are not complete organisms. And even if they were, scientists have found a way to harvest the stem cells without harming the rest of the cells in the blastocyst.

Dr. Ronald Green, Professor for the Study of Ethics and Human Value at Dartmouth College and Chair for the Ethic Advisory Board for Advanced Cell Technology, was featured in a discussion on AirTalk public radio station KPCC-FM in the Los Angeles area. Dr. Green revealed that a way had been found to grow new lines of stem cells from a single cell of a blastocyst. Arnold Kriegstein, M.D., Ph.D, neural stem cell researcher and director of the UCSF Institute for Regeneration Medicine, was also featured on the radio program. Kriegstein affirmed that the removal of a single cell from a blastocyst can be done without harming the rest of the blastocyst. The report was confirmed in *Nature* journal by researchers from a biotechnology firm in Alameda, California. The claim is supported by the fact that thousands of healthy children who began as *in vitro* clusters had pre-implantation genetic diagnosis performed prior to implantation. The diagnosis was done to assure parents that a diseased gene (known to be carried by one parent) was not reproduced in their offspring.

In pre-implantation genetic diagnosis, one cell is removed from an 8- to 16-cell blastocyst for testing purposes. It is allowed to multiply/divide overnight. One of the three new cells is examined the next morning. If it is free of the diseased gene, the rest of the blastocyst is introduced to the uterus where it can begin to successfully produce a healthy baby. The remaining two cells that were grown can then be used to create new stem cell lines by simply allowing them to continue growing. However, these new lines would not be eligible for the NIH registry for federal funding since they were created after the August 2001 cut off imposed by the Bush Administration.

Since no fertilized eggs need to be destroyed, this knowledge could have relieved our president's hesitancy to allow federal funding for IV-B stem cells and remove the cut off date. It did not change his mind because the research that led to the discovery of pre-implantation genetic diagnosis destroyed blastocysts before scientists successfully learned how to do the procedure. Bush stood firm in his position and led others to do the same.

Folks don't seem to be upset about the diseased or unused blastocysts being discarded, or they would be targeting *in vitro* fertilization clinics like they do abortion clinics. If an embryo is being destroyed by research, what is happening to those being thrown in the trash? Aren't they being murdered as well? If a person really believes that human babies are being destroyed through IV-B research, surely they would never participate in *in vitro* fertilization and allow the "murder" of their unused embryos. In fact, they would be trying to stop all *in vitro* fertilization. However, to deny *in vitro* procedures would be to deny life to "snowflake" babies. Maybe President Bush should offer tax incentives to women who adopt and implant leftover blastocysts.

Snowflake Children

If this valuable research material is not going to be used for implantation in hopes of conception, the cells could be used to allow surrogacy childbirth. I have a friend who is the mother of a child she never carried in her womb. Karen participated in an oocyte (egg) donor program. While it is not normal to know who receives donated ova or sperm, Karen did. She had a desire to help her friends Sam and Jody—a married couple who could not have children. Karen's eggs were fertilized *in vitro* by Sam's sperm, then implanted into Jody's womb where she conceived and gave birth to a healthy baby named Rylan. Karen is a regular part of her surrogate son's life. In fact, Karen's natural son, Mack, is her surrogate son's playmate. Babies born to surrogate parents who adopted them as *in vitro* blastocysts are sometimes called "snowflake" children.

However, not all leftover blastocysts are going to be adopted and birthed by surrogate mothers. Most are going to be placed into a red biohazard bag and thrown in the trash. If the owners of cells created *in vitro* are not going to use them and are willing to donate them for research purposes, scientists should be allowed to use them to further the research process. Nearly half of infertile couples say they would like to see some good come from their excess eggs. The fate of these cells has already been decided within the measure of the law and there is no opportunity for a living soul to inhabit those cells. Cells do not care whether they create one organ or an entire human being. Cells simply want to make new cells; it's what they do!

The *in vitro* process unites cells that create more cells.

"Cells, cells, nothing but cells, that's what stem cell research is all about," says Don C. Reed, a board member of the campaign for Proposition 71, California's $3 billion stem cell act.

It's not only ignorant to assume that embryos are produced by IVF, it is anti-woman. Women are more than egg machines. No baby can be produced outside a woman's body. A blastocyst can only become an embryo inside a woman's womb because conception and implantation are required in order for the blastocyst to advance to the stage of an embryo. Those who believe there are embryos in a Petri dish leave out the importance of a woman's role in child bearing.

What's Freezing in the Lab?

There are no unused embryos in a fertility clinic; there are sperm, ova, and fertilized eggs at stages of zygote, morula, and blastocyst development. These cells are on deposit at clinics for the purpose of future use to ensure that a couple who is now fertile will still be able to have children when they are older. For example, some prescription medications and medical procedures can cause sterility. If someone is going to have chemotherapy, or some other procedure that could render him or her sterile, they are wise to make a deposit at a lab which offers cryopreserve storage. Their sperm and ova can be united and frozen until the couple is ready to become pregnant. At that time the fertilized cells will be implanted into a woman's healthy womb where conception may occur and normal gestation may proceed.

If a couple decides that they do not want to have children after utilizing *in vitro* services, they may not want to continue paying the lab to hold their deposits. In such cases, those unused blastocysts are going to be discarded. In my opinion, this disposal of cells is no more inhumane than the body's natural method of disposing of sperm or ova either through the menstrual cycle or by douching after sexual intercourse. Using leftover IV-Bs for research is about as heartless as flushing a tampon and should have the same moral consideration.

Chapter Six

WHAT DOES CLONING HAVE TO DO WITH STEM CELL RESEARCH?

Thirty years ago, new advances in DNA technology led some people to believe that cloning would create cloned humans to be used for body parts. Movies such as *The Island* and *The Boys From Brazil*, and *The 6th Day* have not helped the public understand the benefits of cloning. Rather than creating designer babies, the technology of cloning has led to the development of a biotech industry that has created drugs and diagnostic tests for dozens of diseases. This industry generates billions of dollars in annual revenues which is an advantage for any modern society.

Cloning is the creation of multiple copies of a single molecule, cell, or virus. Cloning is not a new idea. Twins occur naturally when a fertilized egg splits and forms two separate identities. Many people think that cloning and stem cell research are the same thing. They are not. Both cloning and research are procedures that are done with stem cells. Research can be done on stem cells without cloning them; however, cloning a stem cell creates multiple new cells upon which research may be performed reducing the need for new donor material. That is particularly important in light of the limitations the Bush Administration has placed upon federally funded research. There are several hundred thousand leftover frozen blastocysts created after August 2001 in IVF clinics around the country, which could be used for research and to generate new stem cell lines. More IVF-derived blastocysts are added every time a couple opts to utilize IVF to assist with conception, and scientists need them desperately. The sixty lines of preexisting IV-B stem cell lines approved by the Bush Administration represent only a few genetic backgrounds and many are unusable for research purposes. Why anyone believes it's morally and ethically superior to discard IV-B stem cells in a biomedical trash bag rather than use them to find cures that could save human lives is beyond me. But, many people believe what they are told, and even our president has lied to people.

On April 10, 2002, President Bush gave a speech on human cloning legislation through the White House Press Office stating:

> *I believe all human cloning is wrong, and both forms of cloning ought to be banned, for the following reasons. First, anything other than a total ban on human cloning would be unethical. Research cloning would contradict the most fundamental principle of medical ethics, that no human life should be exploited or extinguished for the benefit of another. Yet a law permitting research cloning, while forbidding the birth of a cloned child, would require the destruction of nascent human life.*[27]

From President Bush's statement we see two things: there are two types of cloning, and he believes both should be banned. What scientific fact did he use to support his opinion in the above statement? Obviously, he does not understand the difference in the two types of laboratory cloning.

Types of Laboratory Cloning

Cloning is a very useful tool in all types of research. Powerful new drugs, insulin, and useful bacteria are produced in the lab through cloning. Researchers are able to produce new plants and livestock and track the origins of biological weapons through the cloning process. Cloning is very important to research of stem cells. However, to be used for a specific individual, stem cells need to be modified to genetically match the patient's DNA to avoid being rejected by the body's immune system. This problem can be solved through cloning.

There are two ways to clone or create a cell: 1) Altered Nuclear Transfer (ANT) and Somatic Cell Nuclear Transfer (SCNT), which are also known as therapeutic cloning; 2) Human reproductive cloning, which would utilize the same technique as that used to clone Dolly the sheep.

Both types of cloning start with two cells: one will be an unfertilized egg cell (ova) from which the woman's DNA has been removed from the nucleus. These are called blank cells or empty eggs. The other cell is one that has no ability to reproduce itself such as a skin cell from an adult patient. The DNA from the skin cell is extracted and placed into the empty egg in a Petri dish. Electricity (not fertilization) is used to kick start the cell division process. SCNT and ANT involves no sperm, no implantation in the womb, no womb, and absolutely no embryo. ANT is a supposedly-different version of SCNT, but it is still "nuclear transfer."

After the egg cell begins to divide, it forms a cluster of cells known as a blastocyst. Five to six days later, inner stem cells from this cluster are separated into individual cells and placed into a culture dish. Apart from one another these cells are unable to develop into an entire organism. Biologists then attempt to coax these separate undifferentiated cells to continue to divide into more undifferentiated, pluripotent cells. As a result, an embryonic stem cell line is created. This process is called therapeutic cloning. Human reproductive cloning differs from therapeutic cloning. With reproductive cloning the blastocyst is kept intact and may be implanted in a uterus of an animal and brought to term.

The term Altered Nuclear Transfer (ANT) was proposed by Bush Bioethics Council member and Stanford professor William Hurlbut. Essentially, Hurlbut proposes that scientists first inactivate a gene required for development beyond blastocyst stage. If the correct gene is picked, then it would be possible to generate an altered, cloned blastocyst that has pluripotent stem cells in it. But, because the critical gene is inactive, the blastocyst cannot grow to become an embryo, and thus could not become human. Hurlbut proposed this as an "ethical" way to advance SCNT research.

Don Reed, Chair, Californians for Cures and board officer of Americans for Stem Cell Therapies and Cures, gives a description of nuclear transfer that makes it sound like a pretty simple procedure:

> *What is nuclear transfer? Take a Q-tip®, swab out the inside of the patient's cheek. That gives you a microscopic skin cell. Now add that to an egg like a woman loses every month. Put it in a dish of salt water. Shock it with electricity. Wait 5-7 days, and take it apart. There are your stem cells. No sperm, no implantation in the womb, no womb, and absolutely no child—except maybe the patient being healed. The advantages of having cells to heal—that would not be rejected by the body? Enormous.*[28]

RIGHT TO RECOVER—*Yvonne Perry*

By using one stem cell from an IV-B, researchers can create millions of additional stem cells of the same type. For example, if a blank egg cell is united with the DNA from a person's kidney cells, the result will be the creation of duplicate kidney cells containing the exact DNA of the donor. The cloned kidney cells will not grow a heart, lung, or other organ cells. This type of cloning is useful whenever many cells are needed at one time, as when doctors need to grow a patch of skin for a patient who has suffered a severe burn. These SCNT cloned stem cells may be used to replace a missing element or a dysfunctional cell, but they cannot be used to create an entire human being *in vitro*.

Scientists have been learning how to clone certain body parts (i.e.: an internal organ) through SCNT. Being able to grow rejection-free transplant tissue and organs would be an incredible breakthrough in science and medicine. But don't worry about them creating a Frankenstein using SCNT. Even if science cloned every organ, tissue, blood vessel, muscle, nerve, bone, etc. in the human body, the parts would still have to be assembled perfectly and made to function as a whole.

Those who are opposed to cloning and blastocystic stem cell research may be thinking that reproductive cloning may produce an entire human being designed in a manner that causes original humans to be considered inferior. It's true that we could take a cloned blastocyst, place it into a uterus and allow it to move forward through the stages of gestation and be brought to full-term. That is what scientists did in 1996 to clone Dolly the lamb from a single mammary cell of an adult sheep to create an almost perfect clone. However, it was no easy task. It took 42 attempts before one Dolly was born. Scientists have also created dogs, cats, horses, donkeys, cows, pigs, rabbits, mice, rats, and goats, but no primates. Reproductive cloning can be done, but it may not be biologically possible with humans. Human DNA is much more finicky and the molecular structure of human eggs is easily damaged during cloning. Additionally, human cloning has serious ethical and social implications since we do not know the results such experiments might return. What would be the fate of a severely deformed scientifically-created human? What if an experiment produced an illness that could be hereditarily transmitted to future generations? I do not support or see the need for reproductive cloning in humans. However, I do support SCNT cloning due to its enormous therapeutic value.

President Bush said he would sign a federal bill known as Brownback-Landrieu Senate bill and H.R. 2505 that would make SCNT a felony, punishable by ten years in jail and a fine of $1 million.

"Government policies have to change. We cannot allow such extreme positions to rule the day. Stem cell biology promises to revolutionize the practice of medicine," said Dr. John A. Kessler, Boshes professor and chairman of the Davee Department of Neurology at Northwestern University's Feinberg School of Medicine. "Every real stem cell biologist has no interest in doing reproductive cloning. Make that illegal. That's no problem. Just don't stop us from doing this (therapeutical cloning), because this technique will allow us to generate designer stem cells that could be used to regenerate faulty organs."

Unlike our current president, former presidents understood the value of SCNT cloning. Former President Jimmy Carter stated in a letter to President Bush:

> *...One of the great scientific accomplishments of our time, therapeutic cloning or nuclear transplantation, (SCNT) presents*

promising new opportunities for the treatment of many serious illnesses and injuries that have long plagued the world. These include heart disease, Parkinson's, and spinal cord injury just to name a few. …Though I fully support banning reproductive cloning, I strongly oppose any restrictions on therapeutic cloning.[29]

The Late Former President Gerald Ford once said:

Therapeutic cloning or nuclear transplantation may have enormous potential for the treatment of heart disease, diabetes, Alzheimer's disease, Parkinson's, spinal cord injury and a vast array of other disease and injuries. Unlike reproductive cloning, this approach will never produce a cloned human being. But it could result in the development of life-saving therapies that could improve the well-being of all Americans…Allowing recombinant DNA research to proceed produced significant advances in the prevention and treatment of diseases and illnesses that affect millions of Americans including vaccines, insulin for diabetics and treatments for AIDS and cancer… I strongly urge you to use the recombinant DNA model as a precedent, and allow research conducted for therapeutic purposes to proceed.[30]

SCNT research is supported by the American Medical Association (AMA), the National Academy of Sciences, the Association of American Universities, many communities of faith and national women's rights groups, Nancy Reagan, Gerald Ford, Jimmy Carter, the late Christopher Reeve, Michael J. Fox, more than 40 Nobel laureates, the Coalition for the Advancement of Medical Research (representing more than 80 patient's rights and disease advocacy groups)—and every major medical, scientific, and educational group that has taken a position on the issue. Yet, President Bush believes a total ban on cloning is needed.

RIGHT TO RECOVER—*Yvonne Perry*

To ban SCNT cloning would be a major step backwards for humankind—especially in the U.S. It will be to everyone's advantage if the person elected as president in 2008 has a more scientific understanding of cloning and stem cell research. Hopefully, that person will have no tendency to be swayed by religious myths.

What are the Disadvantages of Cloning?

There are federal restrictions to keep scientists from experimenting using humans, but animal subjects are allowed. Cultured stem cells have the capacity for enormous benefit if their growth and differentiation can be controlled, but they also have significant capacity for harm if that growth and differentiation is not controlled and they cause disease. Cultured stem cells often perform badly and do not always produce the desired cell products.

The animals that have been cloned are subject to premature aging and other health-related complications. Dolly the lamb, named after singer Dolly Parton, was euthanized in 2003 due to lung disease. Ian Wilmut, the scientist whose team at Scotland's Roslin Institute cloned Dolly, opposes the cloning of human beings, citing it as "pointless and cruel."

So, what is the purpose of producing cloned animals? Animals can be genetically altered before they are born to produce proteins in their milk that may be used as drugs to treat humans. The term "pharming" has been given to the science of designing animals for pharmaceutical purposes. I'm not sure I trust the government enough to knowingly eat meat from cloned animals. Scientific discoveries need to be tested over time and not on humans. While we need to devote our energy and resources to conquering disease,

I underscore the need for ethical and social monitoring as cloning technology develops.

Another purpose for cloning is to help researchers learn about the behavior of stem cells in order to discover how degenerative conditions may be reversed. Scientists hope it will one day heal damaged bodies by rejuvenating tissue. They also hope to recreate organs for transplant; to rebuild broken spinal cords and restore nervous systems and brains. Animal studies thus far have shown rejection rates are greatly reduced when a rat receives a transplant of its own DNA. The purpose of this type of cloning is to possibly discover a way to grow human parts in an animal. For example, growing a pig with a human pancreas might be used to derive islet cells for transplantation in a human with diabetes.

Now that you have a better understanding of ANT and SCNT, you will be able to make an informed decision should your state allow you to vote on legislation regarding cloning.

Chapter Seven

NATIONAL RESEARCH

President Bush may have put a lid on federal efforts to advance blastocyst stem cell research, but this did not stop individual states from putting pressure on elected officials to expand the research. In fact, a candidate's position on the topic was a major influence in the outcomes in November 2006's Governor, Senator, and Representative elections. Elected officials from some states gave substantial private funds to independent IV-B research labs to push stem cell and public health initiatives through. Ballots in California, Colorado, Connecticut, Florida, Illinois, Maryland, Missouri, New Jersey, and Wisconsin contained legislation regarding stem cell research to be funded by the state government.

United States

Regardless of what is true at the federal level, many of the American States support blastocystic research. As many as 25 states place some type of restriction on the research, but Indiana, Arkansas, Iowa, Michigan, North and South Dakota ban human cloning for any purpose including therapeutic research. Some states passed bills having restrictions on research procedures while allocating state dollars to be used for IV-B stem cell research. Connecticut, California, New Jersey, Maryland, and Massachusetts passed legislation supporting IV-B stem cell science with strict oversight. Only Massachusetts did not allocate any state funds for the research.

Major universities in each of the fifty states have some type of biomedical research lab and many are working with stem cells. State laws on the issue vary widely: some allow SCNT cloning, some allow research on fetuses and IV-Bs, Louisiana prohibits research on IV-Bs and South Dakota strictly forbids research on IV-Bs regardless of the source. Some states still battle on what is considered a human being and whether or not it includes blastocysts, embryos or fetuses. Other states disagree on what type of research should be funded with public money.

Keeping up with the rapidly changing legislation for stem cell research in each state would be a full time job. More than likely, by the time this manuscript is published some of the material will already be obsolete. In order to keep this book moving along, I will only highlight the research conducted in states that have made a major contribution to IV-B stem cell research through private or public funds. Below is a summary of activities for these states.

California

Of all states in America, California has taken the most aggressive action to support and provide funding for stem cell research. In November 2004, the California Institute for

Regenerative Medicine (CIRM) in San Francisco was established when the voters of California overwhelmingly approved the passage of Proposition 71, also known as the California Stem Cell Research and Cures Act. Proposition 71 establishes a state constitutional right to pursue stem cell research, including SCNT. Over a ten year period, Proposition 71 is projected to provide about $3 billion in stem cell research ($350 million per year over a 10-year period). The purpose of CIRM is to fund research that will support ongoing studies of pluripotent and progenitor cells by scientists who have a record of accomplishment in the field. The intent is to bring new investigators into the research field.

CIRM initiated the sale of bond anticipation notes (BANs) with treasurer approval. That led to $14 million in training grants in 2005. California Governor Arnold Schwarzenegger, a strong supporter of stem cell research, diverted a $150 million loan from the State's General Fund. The BANs funding the research were purchased by private individuals and philanthropic foundations.

CIRM, governed by the Independent Citizens Oversight Committee (ICOC), will evaluate the scientific merit of each grant proposal it receives. It had received more than 200 proposals from researchers at 36 California non-profit institutions as of October 2006. The board made funding recommendations to the full committee to award grant monies raised through bond anticipation notes. The funds now available for use in California equal nearly half the entire national funding received from the NIH for IV-B stem cell research in 2003. The ICOC may award up to $24 million for 30 Scientific Excellence through Exploration and Development (SEED) Grants. Unfortunately, Prop 71 is tied up in red tape litigation with abortion foes and anti-tax advocates. It may be another year before CIRM has access to its general obligation bond capacity. With a requirement that those seeking funds from these agencies obtain matching funds from other sources, the state of California is well on its way to becoming the blastocystic stem cell research hub of the world.

Dr. Hans Kierstead, associate professor at University of California, Irvine is considered one of the foremost researchers of stem cells and their uses. He is the scientist who figured out how to turn blastocyst stem cells into brain cells (oligodendrocytes) that form the insulation around neurons and carry the signals that relay sensations to the brain and tell muscles to move. He and his team of scientists used a treatment based on human IV-B stem cells to greatly improve the gait of a spinal cord injured rat.

Proposition 71 advocate Don Reed has a son named Roman who was paralyzed in a college football accident ten years ago. The Roman Reed Spinal Cord Injury Research Act, "Roman's law" has gathered more than $40 million to research geared toward the cure of paralysis. At an October 24, 2006, press conference Don said:

> *On March 1, 2002, I held in my hands a laboratory rat which had been paralyzed, but which now walked again. It had been given human embryonic stem cells. I felt the tiny muscles moving—muscles which had been still and limp before—and this while my paralyzed son watched from his wheel chair.*
>
> *That research must go forward.*
>
> *Unfortunately there are politicians in Washington who use their power not to help, not to heal—but to just get in the way.*

RIGHT TO RECOVER—*Yvonne Perry*

People like George Bush. People like Richard Pombo.

George Bush refused to sign a very modest little bill called the Stem Cell Research Enhancement Act, such a cautious and careful bill that it passed both the Republican-dominated House and Senate. That bill would have allowed stem cells to be made from biological materials left over from in vitro fertility procedures— blastocysts that were going to be thrown away. These would have been exactly like the stem cell lines made before August 9, 2001, which Mr. Bush approved. The only difference was the date.

But George Bush vetoed that bill, the only veto of his six long years in office. These cells, those few microscopic cells, were judged to be more important than my paralyzed son.[31]

Even though Dr. Hans Keirstead was one of the leading scientific voices behind the movement that persuaded California voters to adopt Proposition 71, he doesn't plan to use public funds for his research. Instead, he is working with Geron Corporation—a biotechnology company in Menlo Park, California that is providing about $500,000 a year to Dr. Keirstead's lab. As a result, Geron holds some of the fundamental patent rights.

Dr. Keirstead, and Dr. Thomas B. O'Karma, President of Geron, plan to launch clinical trials to check for safety in humans next year. The oligodendrocytes derived from stem cells would be inserted into the spinal columns of patients during surgery that commonly follows spinal cord injury. Geron will have to apply to the Food and Drug Administration and receive approval before beginning the trial.

The December 19, 2000, issue of *Proceedings of the National*

RIGHT TO RECOVER—*Yvonne Perry*

Academy of Sciences reported that the University of California Irvine College of Medicine (UCI) had injected a naturally occurring peptide called Transforming Growth Factor-alpha (TGF-Alpha) into damaged areas of rat brains modeling Parkinson's disease. TGF-Alpha (also called GFA-50) stimulates the stem cells already in the brain to multiply, migrate to the locus of damage, and differentiate into fully functional replacement neural and glial cells. Injections of TGF-Alpha into normal rat brain tissue did not stimulate growth of new cells, so the peptide appears to repair damage but not to cause unwanted cell growth. It seems the cells have a "mind" of their own and know exactly what needs to be fixed and what doesn't. It is hoped that these results can be replicated in humans to repair damaged brains and restore function for people with neurological diseases and injuries such as stroke, spinal cord damage, Parkinson's, and Alzheimer's.

Findings from this study conducted by UCI anatomy and neurobiology professor Dr. James Fallon and his colleagues were presented by NIH to the U.S. Congress to show that mobilization of adult neural stem cells is a promising method to treat neurological disorders and brain injury. While no one yet has any approved and effective therapeutic for existing central nervous system damage, Dr. Fallon's work with Transforming Growth Factor-alpha holds great promise and is certainly far too important to ignore.

Dr. Fallon serves as the Chief Science Officer at Neurorepair, Inc., founded and funded by entrepreneur Matthew Klipstein. Neurorepair, Inc. is dedicated to finding a way to repair central nervous system damage. Even though Neurorepair's experiments are still quite preliminary, the company is not alone in its belief that stimulating the body's own adult stem cells to affect repair (as opposed to transplanting foreign stem cells) is likely to be a better approach. Stem Cell Therapeutics of Calgary, Canada is also working on a method of stimulating proliferation of one's own adult stem cells to heal the brain. However, Stem Cell Therapeutics is concentrating on a therapeutic window of just a few hours, while Neurorepair is trying to develop something that may be effective months or even years after an injury has stabilized.

Dr. Evan Snyder is a pediatrician and neurologist. He left his practice at Harvard Medical School to further his work in the field of stem cell biology at Burnham Institute in California when he saw that California was beginning to lead the world in stem cell research.

Burnham Institute is forging ahead as a pioneer in fundamental biology—a branch of developmental biology that studies the behavior of stem cells and makes application to what diseases they might treat. Both privately and federally funded, Burnham uses all kinds of stem cells for study; human, animal, IV-B, blood cord, fetus, bone marrow, and placenta. Presently, Burnham is conducting tests on large primates to treat Parkinson's disease. Dr. Snyder describes a stem cell as the most immature, primordial cell of the nervous system.

> *Think of it almost like the smart seeds of the brain. These seeds are the kind of seeds that if you throw them on the lawn, they know to become grass, but if they land in a flower bed they also know to become tulips or roses or daffodils. So it's like reseeding the lawn with really smart seeds. If we can understand how these seeds work, how to obtain them, disburse them, and get them to become*

*what we want them to become, then we can use this knowledge for
a whole range of diseases such as Alzheimer's disease, Parkinson's
disease, or even acquired conditions like head injury, stroke, and
spinal-cord injury.*[32]

Dr. Snyder was the first to isolate and grow neural stem cells
in the lab about ten years ago. His method is licensed to Layton
Bioscience Inc. of Atherton, California, which plans to develop
stem cell treatments. Dr. Snyder's neural stem cell research was
conducted on cells originally taken from a fetus that was aborted
several years ago.

Dr. Evan Snyder has gained national prominence in the field
of stem cell biology. He is constantly flying from one scientific
meeting to another, writing papers, supervising his laboratory,
and keeping in touch with countless scientists with whom he's
collaborating. His desire to find a cure for a wide range of presently
incurable brain disorders led him to focus on creating tissue from
stem cells that can be used as human donor material. He says, "If
scientists can perfect their knowledge of what flips on the switch
to make embryonic stem cells branch off to become a particular
tissue type, they can direct the stem cells to be the tissue required
to treat a patient."

Within a couple of years, Dr. Snyder hopes that human
neural stem cells can be administered to animal models through
a fairly simple delivery system which will allow these cells to find
their proper place in the brain. Once there, he hopes they will live,
become the appropriate missing cells, and send out and find the
appropriate target and start functioning, and that they'll do this
in a very safe and effective manner. He says, "We're getting to the

point where the obstacle is no longer the biology, the obstacle is the lack of resources. With enough resources, we could start working around the clock. The quicker we work, the quicker the data becomes available, the quicker we can troubleshoot, fix it, and then start putting together a story that would be approved by a regulatory commission."

Dr. Snyder implanted neural stem cells into the brain of a lab mouse afflicted with continuous, severe tremors. The implanted cells repaired the damage and eased the mouse's shaking. Dr. Snyder has also done this type of stem cell work with monkeys, since they more closely resemble humans.

> *We're progressing at a pace that is every scientist's dream, but it's very important not to sacrifice our scientific integrity in the rush toward a cure. Nor can the research move into humans before the safety of stem cells is known. We have to know if these things can be controlled once they're implanted. In addition, the Food and Drug Administration will want assurance that the versatile cells won't produce cancers, and that the cells can be produced with consistent quality control.*[33]

Dr. Snyder is dedicated to solving childhood disorders through blastocyst stem cells, and his true passion is in finding a cure for rare disorders in kids and pre-mature babies. Rather than make mistakes on children, Dr. Snyder uses a limited number of monkeys to test his research. Once he and his team have worked out the kinks and figured out the limitations and the potential of neural stem cells, they hope to be able to at least think about doing clinical trials in some of the pediatric neurological population with severe diseases in which patients have a short life span, no available treatments, and a homogeneous population. These are the only ones likely to be approved by the FDA for early developmental therapies of this technology.

Klein Financial Corporation is a real estate investment banking consulting company of which Robert N. Klein, II is president. Mr. Klein, a Democratic attorney, has a keen interest in stem cell research for personal reasons. His youngest son, Jordan, was diagnosed with Juvenile diabetes in 2001, his mother has Alzheimer's, and his father died from heart disease. Klein served as Committee Chairman of the California Proposition 71 ballot initiative. Klein not only gives his own money to blastocyst stem cell research, he has also been able to raise funds from other philanthropists.

The Reeve-Irvine Research Center for Spinal Cord Injury at the University of California, Irvine (UCI) was named for actor Christopher Reeve. The center was established to study injuries to, and diseases of, the spinal cord and develop strategies to promote repair and regeneration of nerve cells. Professor of Anatomy and Neurobiology Dr. Oswald Steward is the chair and director of the center and serves on the board of the Christopher Reeve Paralysis Foundation and also serves as the chair of its Science Advisory Council. Dr. Steward is the recipient of many research awards for his research on nerve cell behavior, regeneration, growth and function, and how physiological activity affects nerve cell connections. Nerve damage is an illness to hopefully benefit from blastocyst stem cell therapy.

CyThera, Inc. in San Diego, California has produced a solution that spurs blastocyst stem cells to develop into endoderm—a layer that gives rise to the thyroid, thymus, lungs, liver, pancreas, and the lining of the respiratory and digestive tracts. Emmanuel Baetge of CyThera explained, "If you were to use human embryonic stem cells to make products that treat disease, such as diabetes or liver failure, you'd have to go through the endoderm stage to get to it." By using stem cells to generate an unlimited supply of islet cells that produce insulin, there is new hope for treating diabetes.

The University of California in San Francisco (UCSF) is also interested in brain stem cells. Their scientists have determined through a study in mice that a protein called HIPK2 is essential for the survival of dopamine neurons. These are the cells lost in Parkinson's disease. Therapy is being developed for the molecular pathway in which the protein functions. Since mice and humans have the same cells in their brains, it may be possible to treat brain tissues damaged by stroke and traumatic injury. Prominent researchers affiliated with UCSF are Eric J. Huang, M.D., Ph.D; Chay T. Kuo, M.D., Ph.D; Yuh-Nung Jan, Ph.D; Arnold Kriegstein, M.D., Ph.D; Renee Reijo Pera, Ph.D; and Elena Gates, M.D.

Colorado

Because President Bush halted federal funding for new stem cell lines, private investors seeking to advance research on IV-B stem cells are picking up the slack.

Through a $6 million gift to the University of Colorado Health Sciences Center from the Charles C. and June S. Gates Family Fund, Colorado will create the Charles C. Gates Regenerative Medicine and Stem Cell Biology Program. The program will led by Dennis

Roop, Ph.D, a professor and director of the Center for Cutaneous Molecular Biology at Baylor College of Medicine, Houston, Texas. Dr. Roop plans to bring in 34 researchers and five grants from NIH worth about $3.8 million with him when he takes the position as the Chairperson in January 2007.

Since 1988, Dr. Curt Freed, director of the neuro-transplantation program for Parkinson's disease at the University of Colorado Health Sciences Center, and his team (John Sladek and Mike Zawada) have transplanted dopamine cells to ease the suffering of their patients. They use neuronal stem cells derived from animal or human fetuses to repair brain injury. The team never encouraged a woman to end her pregnancy; they simply utilized a by-product of a legal medical procedure for a much higher calling. These fetuses were about to be thrown in the trash.

Congresswoman Diana DeGette of Colorado is a staunch supporter of blastocyst stem cell research. Ms. DeGette is part of a coalition that passed the bill in the House over the objections of GOP leaders, Bush, and social conservatives. She co-sponsored H.R. 810 (the Stem Cell Research Enhancement Act) with Representative Mike Castle. Together they reintroduced the bill as "H.R. 3 in 110th Congress. Her campaign for office was assisted by actor Michael J. Fox—a victim of Parkinson's.

Connecticut

On June 15, 2005, the Connecticut legislature passed Senate Bill 934 "An Act Permitting Stem Cell Research and Banning the Cloning of Human Beings," which created a fund to provide $100 million dollars in state-funded grants a year over a 10-year period.

Approved by the General Assembly of Connecticut and signed by Governor M. Jodi Rell, the passage of this legislation made Connecticut the third state in the U.S. to provide public funding in support of blastocystic and adult stem cell research.

The legislation is being implemented through the development of collaborative relationships which include:

- Office of Research and Development within the Department of Public Health.

- Local, national and international stem cell research community of scientists, policy makers, and advocates.

- Connecticut Innovations (created by the Connecticut Legislature in 1989) to provide capital and operational insight to the biotechnology industry. By helping companies research, develop, and market new products and services, CI has brought in more than $1 billion dollars in additional investments from the private sector. CI has brought the State of Connecticut over $510 million in Gross State Profit and over 5,000 additional job-years.

- Connecticut Stem Cell Research Committee.

- Connecticut United for Research Excellence (CURE), an educational and business support organization that works closely with lawmakers, policy makers, and government officials. With over 100 members including major pharmaceutical companies, emerging biotechnology companies, and major research universities, CURE is keeping Connecticut competitive in bioscience.

- Academic research institutions.

Connecticut is using 95% of their public dollars to support

adult stem cell research and only 5% for blastocystic stem cell research.

Florida

Two state constitutional amendments are being proposed to Florida's 2008 voters. Governor Charlie Crist's proposal calls for research using only stem cells derived from adults, umbilical-cord blood or amniotic fluid, but not *in vitro* blastocysts. The other voter ballot initiative proposal, if passed, will amend the state's constitution to provide state funding ($200 million over 10 years) for blastocyst stem cell research.

Florida residents Faye Armitage and her 16-year-old son, Jason, have been on the stem cell battle field for the ten years since Jason had a collision on a soccer field which left him paralyzed from the nose down.

Faye has lobbied lawmakers from Tallahassee to Washington to promote funding for blastocyst stem cell research. She has opposed unfair constitutional amendments, fought for wheelchair ramps in public schools, waved signs, marched in rallies, driven across the country to visit legislators, written letters, blogged, contributed to several Web sites that are pro-blastocyst stem cell research, and talked to anyone who would listen. She says the right to recover is the next civil-rights movement and is not ashamed that her efforts have landed her in jail twice.

Faye believes that stem cells harvested from *in vitro* fertilized eggs have the best chance of freeing her son and millions of others from life-threatening/diminishing maladies. "I think it's controversial to oppose it. I actually think it's criminal," she said. "I have been called a baby killer many times, but to me the opponents are the ones killing the babies—real babies with real diseases in need of real treatments—not fertilized egg cells that are going to be thrown away. To me . . . we're recycling medical waste."[34]

As a Florida resident, she is also trying to rewrite the language of the Florida debate and hopes Florida will vote to lift the state's current restrictions on IV-B stem cell research. With Jason at her side, Faye volunteers with a grass-roots organization Cure Paralysis Now and spends her weekends collecting signatures for the first petition.

Georgia

The Saving the Cure Act (SB 148) proposed by the Georgia State Senate contains scientifically inaccurate claims that could hinder the progress of IV-B stem cell research in that state. Any effort to disseminate negative and incorrect information about IV-B stem cell research throws unnecessary obstacles in the path of progress and research. CAMR President, Sean Tipton, urges Georgians to write their legislators and ask them to oppose the bill. The bill's purpose to promote cord blood research in Georgia is well and good. However, the preamble section of the bill, also called the "findings," suggests that IV-B stem cell research is failing to lead to cures and can even lead to cancer in patients. While the findings section does not carry the full weight of the law, these false claims are serious enough for CAMR to oppose the legislation unless and until those findings are changed.

RIGHT TO RECOVER—*Yvonne Perry*

Illinois

The day after President Bush vetoed H.R. 810, Illinois Governor Rod Blagojevich (D) signed an executive order to create the Illinois Regenerative Medicine Institute (IRMI) and provide for grants to medical research facilities for adult and IV-B stem cell research. The $15 million will come from administrative funds already set aside for the state Department of Healthcare and Family Services.

Legislators from predominantly Catholic districts proved essential to defeat IRMI legislation in Springfield. However, despite repeated objections from state legislators, Governor Blagojevich took action to invest in research that may save lives and prevent serious illnesses. Blagojevich believes his decision is more than a sound public health strategy; it's our moral obligation. He said, "The promise of stem cell research is unlimited, and countless lives hang in the balance. It's clear we can't count on the President to support stem cell research, and lawmakers in Springfield have yet to act on a proposal that would provide $100 million over five years for research. So we are doing what we can with the resources we have to fund stem cell research. I'm confident that the seven recipients of this funding will make strides towards curing diseases ranging from diabetes to Alzheimer's."[35]

Seven projects at Illinois universities will share $5 million in new state funding for the life-saving work of stem cell research. Recipients were selected from proposals submitted beforehand to the Illinois Department of Public Health's Illinois Regenerative Medicine Institute (IRMI). Funding was awarded to:

- $1,100,000 – Jasti Rao, University of Illinois College of Medicine, Peoria
- $1,000,000 – Lawrence School, University of Illinois, Urbana-Champaign
- $750,000 – Dengping Yin, University of Illinois, Chicago
- $250,000 – Matthew Stewart, University of Illinois, Urbana-Champaign
- $400,000 – Fei Wang, University of Illinois, Urbana-Champaign
- $400,000 – Sara Becker-Catania, University of Illinois, Chicago
- $1,100,000 – Stuart Adler, Southern Illinois University, Carbondale

Illinois U.S. Senator Barack Obama favors all types of stem cell research. In his statement of support for stem cell research, Senator Obama pleaded with President Bush not to veto H.R. 810:

> *Many men, women and children who are cancer survivors are already familiar with the life-saving applications of adult stem cell research. Patients with leukemia or lymphoma often undergo bone marrow transplants, a type of stem cell transplant, which can significantly prolong life, or permanently get rid of the cancer. This therapy has been used successfully for decades, and is saving lives everyday.*
>
> *Yet this breakthrough has its serious limitations. Adult stem cells, such as those used in bone marrow transplants, can only be collected in small quantities, may not be a match for the patient, and*

have limited ability to transform into specialized cells.

Cord blood, like the kind Ryan used, has limitations as well. If, for example, young Ryan's condition should deteriorate or he should develop another illness, there simply are not enough cord blood cells left for a second use. His mother has told us that the few remaining cells would have to be cloned to get enough cells for future use, or they would have to obtain stem cells from another source.

These and other difficulties are the reasons why scientists have started to explore other types and other sources for stem cells, including embryonic stem cell research.

Embryonic stem cells can be obtained from a number of sources, including in vitro fertilization. At this very moment, there are over 400,000 embryos being stored in over 400 facilities throughout the United States. The majority of these are reserved for infertile couples. However, many of these embryos will go unused, destined for permanent storage in a freezer or disposal. We should expand and accelerate research using these embryos, just as we should continue to explore the viability of adult stem cell use and cord blood use.

All over the country, exciting progress is being made in the area of embryonic stem cell research. At the University of Illinois, they're finding that stem cells have the potential to treat blood disorders, lung diseases, and heart damage.

At Johns Hopkins, researchers were able to use mouse embryonic stem cells to repair damaged nerves and restore mobility in paralyzed rats. One can't help but think that it's a matter of when, not if, this research will be able to one day help those who have lost the ability to walk.

For these reasons, I'm proud to be a long-term supporter of greater stem cell research. While I was a member of the Illinois Senate, I was the chief cosponsor of the Ronald Reagan Biomedical Research Act, which would specifically permit embryonic stem cell research in Illinois, and establish review of this research by the Illinois Department of Public Health.

And I'm proud to be a cosponsor of the stem cell bill before us today. This bill embodies the innovative thinking that we as a society demand and medical advancement requires. By expanding scientific access to embryonic stem cells which would be otherwise discarded, this bill will help our nation's scientists and researchers develop treatments and cures to help people who suffer from illnesses and injuries for which there are currently none. But the bill is not without limits; it requires that scientific research also be subject to rigorous oversight.

I realize there are moral and ethical issues surrounding this debate. But I also realize that we're not talking about harvesting cells that would've been used to create life and we're not talking about cloning humans. We're talking about using stem cells that would have otherwise been discarded and lost forever - and we're talking about using those stem cells to possibly save the lives of millions of Americans. Democrats want this bill to pass. Conservative, pro-life Republicans want this bill to pass. By large margins, the American people want this bill to pass. It is only the White House standing in the way of progress - standing in the way of so many potential cures.[36]

I couldn't have said it better myself. Thank you, Mr. Obama.

Despite objections from blastocyst stem cell opponents and some senators who questioned the state's financial ability to shoulder the burden, the Illinois Senate voted 35-23 in February 2007 to spend state tax dollars on blastocyst stem cell research. The bill (SB4) has to pass the Illinois House in order to make the institute and its grants a part of state law.

Republican supporter Senator Kirk Dillard said, "They go into the public sewer system. I really believe my maker would want me to use these embryos to sustain and improve human life."

Not to be left out of the loop on technology derived from stem cells is the cosmetic industry. A Chicago team at the University of Illinois experimenting with mice has shown that with the right chemical cocktail, stem cells can be persuaded to differentiate into skin, fat, or muscle cells. They believe it may be possible to use a patient's stem cells to make natural and safer implants for cosmetic and reconstructive surgery after breast cancer and to repair facial problems after trauma. Interestingly, initial stem cell funding proposal from State Comptroller, Daniel Rynes, was a "luxury tax" on cosmetic surgeries performed in Illinois at which the cosmetic industry balked.

Kansas

Kansas has more than tornadoes and the Wicked Witch of the West to be afraid of. There are three bills floating in February 2007 that make blastocyst stem cell research a felony in Kansas. The bills, if passed, will make Kansas citizens eligible for a $500,000 fine and prison time should they return to the state having cured their disease in another state—regardless of the fact that the research is federally legal.

Maryland

Backed by overwhelming support from advocates for stem cell research, Senator Paula Hollinger, Delegate Samuel Rosenberg, and House Speaker Mike Busch introduced legislation to fund IV-B stem cell research in Maryland. On March 29, 2006, Maryland's Legislature passed the Stem Cell Research Act of 2006 (House Bill 1/Senate Bill 144), and Governor Robert L. Ehrlich, Jr. (R) signed the bill into law making Maryland the fourth state agreeing to government funding for stem cell research. The legislation stipulates:

- IV-Bs must be voluntarily donated by couples who have completed fertility treatments and who would otherwise discard the leftover cells.
- Research funding will be awarded based on scientific merit as judged by a scientific peer review committee. Doctors have an odd scientific review system that includes in-state scientific administrators.
- SCNT (therapeutic cloning) for research is allowed.
- Reproductive cloning that creates human beings is a criminal act.
- Healthcare practitioners are required to provide infertility patients with the information necessary to make informed and voluntary decisions about their surplus frozen IV-Bs.
- Written consent from donors is required.
- Payment for IV-B donation is prohibited.

RIGHT TO RECOVER—*Yvonne Perry*

This legislation created the Maryland Stem Cell Research Fund, which will provide grants for adult and IV-B stem cell research. The Maryland fiscal year 2007 budget includes $15 million in research grants to university and private-sector researchers seeking treatments for debilitating conditions through stem cells, including those derived from IV-Bs. These grants are to help find cures and treatments for chronic illnesses such as Parkinson's disease, Juvenile diabetes, as well as paralysis and severe burns.

Julie Coons, President of the Tech Council of Maryland, hopes the legislation will foster start-up companies and said, "We have made a major step forward in helping the industry but also in sending a message . . . that we are a player in this field."

Much of the money is expected to flow to researchers at Johns Hopkins University, the University of Maryland, and a few companies in Maryland's biotech sector conducting research on adult stem cells. The C. Michael Armstrong Professor, John D. Gearhart, is a leader in the development and use of human reproductive technologies and in the genetic engineering of cells at Johns Hopkins School of Medicine. He is also the director of the Stem Cell Program for the Institute for Cell Engineering at Hopkins. With a focus on how genes regulate the formation of tissues, one of Dr. Gearhart's goals is to determine the causes of Down's syndrome and related birth defects. Dr. Gearhart believes clinical trials for spinal cord injury, stroke, Parkinson's disease, and heart disease will begin on humans within the next couple of years.

Massachusetts

In the above mentioned states, governors took a pro-active stance in pushing for legislation to fund stem cell research. In Massachusetts, Governor Mitt Romney and long-standing pro-life fundamentalists tried to stop it. With an overwhelmingly 35 to 2 vote in the Senate and 117-37 in the House, legislators defeated the Governor and his anti-stem cell advocates in February 2005. All forms of stem cell research are now allowed in Massachusetts. Home to Harvard University, an international leader in the field, Massachusetts was the only state to pass a law supporting IV-B research without providing state funding.

Speaking of Harvard, there is much stem cell work going on at Harvard Stem Cell Institute (HSCI). Researchers at HSCI and Children's Hospital Boston are beginning experiments using SCNT to create disease-specific stem cell lines using blastocyst stem cells to develop treatments for a wide range of incurable conditions. The series of experiments supported entirely with private funds due to federal restrictions on blastocyst stem cell work has been proven in animals.

Douglas Melton, co-director of the HSCI, and Professor Kevin Eggan, Assistant of the Faculty of Arts and Sciences (FAS) Department of Molecular and Cellular Biology, are each leading a team of researchers. Melton's work focuses on diabetes. Dr. Eggan's work focuses on neurodegenerative diseases, such as ALS. Dr. Eggan is also working with cellular differentiation, which causes the nucleus of an adult cell to return to a totipotent state. This process is called nuclear reprogramming. Harvard University Stem

Cell Institute researcher George Daley focuses on blood disorders and uses SCNT to treat immune deficiency.

While Harvard is leading the way in stem cell research in Massachusetts, new legislation allowed the University of Massachusetts to create an institute for stem cell research and regenerative medicine. One-million dollars of state funds may be used on stem cell biology. Ten-million dollars was appropriated to a fund that will establish a center to promote life sciences research in advanced and applied sciences. This includes, but is not limited to, stem cell research, regenerative medicine, biotechnology, and nanotechnology. The legislation created the Life Sciences Investment Fund to oversee appropriations, allocations, grants, or loans to leverage development and investments in stem cell research and other areas.

Dr. John E. Mayer Jr., at Children's Hospital Boston, is a heart surgeon and tissue engineering pioneer who created heart valves fashioned from stem cells harvested from sheep bone marrow. When implanted in sheep, the valves seem to be working normally. This is an incredible breakthrough for science as well as for the state of Massachusetts. Can you imagine all the patients who could be helped by having transplants of organ parts made from their own DNA? The rejection rate would have to be much lower than traditional transplants from foreign donors—no matter how well matched.

Missouri

Thanks to a state constitution amendment created by the 2006 Missouri Stem Cell Research and Cures Initiative, scientists and institutions may conduct any stem cell research permitted by federal law including blastocyst and SCNT cloning. It prohibits the creation of IV-Bs solely for research purposes.

The Executive Director of the Parkinson Foundation of the Heartland, Meg Duggan, strongly believes we are here to be "thought leaders" who must deliver a deeper understanding of where hope lies for a cure to the PD community. Her organization is, in part, responsible for getting the Kansas Coalition for Lifesaving Cures and the Missouri Coalition for Lifesaving Cures on the ballots. Meg's sister was diagnosed with Parkinson's at age 38 and has fought heroically for 11 years working and raising her girls.

Nebraska

Regarding medical and scientific progress, the state of Nebraska may be making a giant step backward. If the bill (LB700) they are considering actually passes, LB700 would ban reproductive cloning and the creation of blastocysts for stem cell research using SCNT. Violators would be guilty of a Class IV felony, which is punishable by a maximum sentence of five years in prison, a $10,000 fine, or both.

New Jersey

When former Governor James McGreevey signed New Jersey's Stem Cell Bill in January 2004, New Jersey became the second state to approve of using public money to fund human IV-B stem cell research. This allowed research using IV-B stem cells lines prohibited for use with federal funding restrictions. In

December 2005, $5.5 million was appropriated to fund the Stem Cell Research Institute of New Jersey and other institutes that support stem cell research. Research grants were made available through the Commission on Science and Technology for the funding of projects at academic, not-for-profit, and for-profit institutions in the State of New Jersey.

Current Governor Jon Corzine's dream to establish New Jersey as a leader in Stem Cell Research and enable groundbreaking IV-B stem cell research in the state is slowly becoming a reality. On December 18, 2006, the Commission on Science and Technology launched a $10 million New Jersey Stem Cell Research Grant Program, which will provide $7 million for core facilities grants to support human blastocyst stem cell research and $3 million for individual research grants.

Texas

In 2003, two stem cell research bills, one pro-research and one anti-research, were filed in the Texas Legislature. After the legislation to ban IV-B stem cell research was defeated near the end of the session, the loosely-organized advocates from numerous disease groups (diabetes, Parkinson's, MS, spinal cord injury, and others) formed TAMR (Texans for Advancement of Medical Research) to lead the effort to protect all forms of stem cell research in Texas.

In 2005, twelve pro-research bills (ranging from simply protecting IV-B stem cell research from a ban, to protecting the research and constructing ethical guidelines and oversight, to funding all types of stem cell research) were filed, and three anti-research bills. Because state officials at the highest levels threatened to veto any pro-research bill, and TAMR's legislative team succeeded in blocking the anti-research bills, none of the 15 pieces of legislation moved out of committee.

In the 2006 Special Session, funding was again attempted to build a stem cell research center. The Tuition Revenue Bond bill did not contain restrictive language, so an attempt was made to amend it in order to ban IV-B stem cell research. As a compromise, the stem cell research facility was pulled out of the bill.

Parkinson's Action Network (PAN) is a national organization whose primary objective is to educate and advocate for funding for Parkinson's research. Texas State coordinator, Nina Brown, struggles with Parkinson's disease. In 2003, Texas HB 1175 was presented, which would have criminalized blastocyst stem cell research in Texas. This petite, attractive grandmother, along with husband, Joe, made numerous trips to the state capitol to advocate against that bill and other legislation. The effort has proven to be so effective that no bill criminalizing IV-B stem cell research has made it to either house of the Texas legislature.

Another important outcome of the Browns' advocacy efforts was the co-founding of Texans for Advancement of Medical Research (TAMR) in 2003. This organization is composed of scientists, physicians, ethicists, leading health groups, and individuals who support biological research in regenerative medicine.

"Our purpose is to raise public awareness on the issues surrounding regenerative biomedical research. We will continue to educate our public officials in Texas and advocate for all those whose health depends on it. Our organization is inclusive. It consists of Jews, Protestants, Catholics, and all those who believe this is a health issue, not a religious issue," wrote Nina in a document she emailed me.

To further that end, another group focusing on education rather than advocacy, The Alliance for Medical Research (TAMR-ed), was established. As Secretary and a Founding Board Member, Nina co-wrote an excellent explanation of IVF blastocysts and SCNT. TAMR-ed produced the outstanding video "Regenerative Medicine - Pathways to Cures."

New York

For the last three years a coalition of disease advocacy, research institutions, scientists and social organizations and patients (NYAMR—New Yorkers for the Advancement of Medical Research) has been working to pass legislation protecting and funding IV-B stem cell research in New York State through lobbying and educating lawmakers and the public.

During the first two years, the Democratic Assembly passed pro-research bills that died in the Republican controlled Senate. Last year leaders of both houses said they supported stem cell research, but couldn't agree on how to fund it. The former Republican Governor George Pataki probably wouldn't have supported any funding. There's also a politically strong and well-organized Catholic Conference in New York State who oppose any funding for IV-B stem cell research.

New York has a new governor—Eliot Spitzer—a moderate Democrat who says he supports the research. He is proposing a bond issue to fund life sciences research, including IV-Bs with a $2.1 billion 10-year bond issue that would be voted on in 2008.

He's tying research funding with economic development. In 2007, $100 million was included in his budget for 2007-08 to jump start research. NYAMR is trying to work with the governor and legislators to make sure the bill is written so that IV-B research funding can't be challenged in the courts, as they did in California, and so that the funding will go where it is needed most and have the greatest impact.

Wisconsin

Through the efforts of Governor Jim Doyle and the University of Wisconsin School of Medicine and Public Health, Wisconsin is noticed as a pioneer in stem cell research. In 1995, University of Wisconsin (UW) Scientist and Professor of Anatomy, James Thomson, isolated and cultured non-human primate and human blastocyst stem cells and then published his findings in the November 1998 issue of *Science.* Thompson's involvement as the chief pathologist at the Wisconsin National Primate Research Center and the Wisconsin Regional Primate Research Center is marked by his pioneering work and significant breakthroughs.

On October 10, 2006, Governor Jim Doyle announced $1 million in funding for Stem Cell Products, Inc. (SCP), which creates blood products from blastocyst stem cells. SCP was founded by UW James Thomson, Igor Slukvin and Dong Chen and other researchers with the intent of doing commercial research and developing processes to make safe, effective blood products (red blood cells and platelets) from IV-B stem cells. SCP will receive $750,000 in loans and a $250,000 grant from the Wisconsin Department of Commerce to help develop techniques that allow industrial-scale manufacturing of blood products for human clinical use. Governor Doyle speaks highly of the company:

> *This company is an example of the enormous potential of embryonic stem cell research not only to heal illness but to create new, high paying jobs in Wisconsin. I'll continue fighting to make sure that top researchers and embryonic stem cell companies are welcomed with open arms and have the strong support of the state. Their work will save lives, transform our economy and open the doors to the jobs of the future.*[37]

The state's concern is over the ever-increasing cost of treating the symptoms, effects, and conditions of diseases. Wisconsin Stem Cell Now, Inc. says, "When stem cell research uncovers the cause, cures, therapies, and preventative strategies of diseases, healthcare costs will significantly shrink. A cut of simply 1% will pay for itself and reduce healthcare costs by tens of billions of dollars in future decades."

The Wisconsin Institutes for Discovery will receive $375 million to construct world-class twin facilities joined by a central atrium, one public and one private, in the heart of UW-Madison campus beginning in 2008. Both the public institute (Wisconsin Institute for Discovery) and the private institute (Morgridge Institute for Research) are also funded by a $50 million gift from UW-Madison alumni, John and Tasha Morgridge, and matching gifts from WARF and the state of Wisconsin.

Wisconsin vows to conduct research with integrity by stating it is not using human reproductive cloning and promises to never create cloned fetuses.

See http://isscr.org/public/regions/states.cfm#About for

Chapter Eight

INTERNATIONAL RESEARCH

Although the first blastocystic stem cell line was created in the United States, a majority of new lines are now being created overseas, causing America to lose its preeminence in one of the most active areas of biological discovery. American scientists are losing their ability to remain at the cutting edge of research and many are being lured to countries that have more flexible standards.

The countries most advanced in their discoveries are the ones having less religious influence and government restriction. The U.S. lags behind due to opposition from President Bush and some ultra-conservative citizens. This debate not only slows the pace of research that could lead to cures, it also puts the U.S. behind in technologies that would provide new business opportunities.

European Countries

Soon after Bush's veto of a bill intended to expand federal funding for blastocystic stem cell biology in the U.S., the European Union (E.U.) agreed to allow funding for human IV-B stem cell research. In spite of fierce opposition from predominantly Roman Catholic countries (Malta, Lithuania, Poland and Slovakia), the European Parliament voted 300 to 210 to back public funding of research on stem cells extracted from human blastocysts without destroying them. The bloc included a ban on human cloning for reproductive purposes and on research intended to modify the genetic integrity of humans—a particularly sensitive issue in Germany where people still remember Nazi genetic experiments. This decision allowed countries within the E.U. that legalize blastocystic stem cell research to move forward without being held back by conservative countries. The funding of approximately $64 billion (U.S.) will come from the E.U.'s research budget for 2007 to 2013. Individual E.U. countries can decide whether or not to contribute to the funding.

Sweden

Clustered around Karolinska Institute in Stockholm, Sahlgrenska Academy in Gothenburg, and Lund University in southern Sweden, there are more than thirty research groups and 300 people working at nine Swedish institutions.

Research produces treatment and technology. Technology is followed by commercial ventures. As a result of the promising results of Swedish research on IV-B stem cells, several start-up companies have been founded in Stockholm and Gothenburg. These companies hope to reap the financial benefits as they bring to the market any new technology and biomedicine to treat illnesses.

Sweden leads the world in stem cell research most likely because Sweden's government is supportive of all areas of stem cell research, including therapeutic cloning. Here are a few of their accomplishments:

- Göteborg University in Göteborg holds nineteen of the remaining lines of stem cells approved by the Bush Administration that have not been found to be contaminated.

- Groups at the Sahlgrenska University Hospital in Gothenburg led by Professor Lars Hamberger have cultured 30 new stem cell lines from blastocysts.

- Karolinska University Hospital at Huddinge, Stockholm has refined a growth medium for blastocyst stem cells that acts as a human fibroblast—a large flat cell that secretes serum and proteins that form collagen and elastic fibers and the substance between the cells of connective tissue. This allows continued undifferentiated division of individual stem cells derived from the inner cell mass of IV-B without the use of animal feeder cells.

- Founded in 1998 by two leading neuroscientists from Karolinska Institute, Stockholm-based NeuroNova developed VEGF protein—shown to protect motor neurons from dying and to increase life span and motor function—for the treatment of ALS (Lou Gehrig's disease). Their drug development projects are aimed at stimulating processes in the brain that lead to the formation of new neurons. The company hopes to use such cells for transplantation therapy in Parkinson's disease and as a platform for drug discovery.

- Another company named OvaCell has access to six of the Bush-approved stem cell lines listed in the NIH register. Therefore, OvaCell is eligible for U.S. funding for research concentrated on development of cell cultivation and differentiation of stem cells into brain, heart, cartilage, and insulin producing cells to treat SCI, heart problems, and diabetes. With its bio-ethical climate and political support for stem cell research, there will be many more stem cell companies, miraculous discoveries, technologies, and treatments in Sweden.

Israel

Jewish law does not consider a blastocyst as potential life until it is inside the uterus of a woman and conception is affirmed. Therefore IV-B stem cell research is not a controversial issue in Israel. Jewish groups in America hold to this same idea and push for funding for stem cell research, which will increase funds for research abroad. Dr. Shulamit Levenberg, a researcher at the Technion University in Haifa, is an observant Jew who hopes to create lab-manufactured tissues and organs for transplants. "In Israel the attitudes are much more positive," she said. "Here it is not thought of as killing the cells but of using them to save life."

Because Israel relies heavily on grants from abroad (especially U.S. grants), Dr. Binyamin Reubinoff, who heads the Hadassah Embryonic Stem Cell Research Center, is concerned about the affect Bush's veto will have upon progress in the field. Reubinoff said, "It has an influence on scientists and the availability for money for research." Hadassah is one of the world's leaders of stem cell research—second to derive stem cells from human blastocysts. Six of the stem cell lines made available for research using U.S. federal funding were produced by this lab. An experiment conducted by Reubinoff's team, which implanted human stem cells into the brains of rats, showed a reduction of symptoms of Parkinson's disease.

Bar-Ilan University professor Ron Goldstein implanted human IV-B stem cells into chicken embryos to study the early stages of normal cellular development and to better understand how familial dysautonomia (a degenerative genetic disease) works and to test possible treatments. "Once we can produce FD-infected nerve tissue in a Petri dish, we will have a model to understand what is happening on a molecular level," Goldstein told the Forward. "And this model could also be used to test new drug therapies for the disease."[38]

The Hebrew University in Israel is another progressive IV-B stem cell research leader. Dr. Nissim Benvenisty met with U.S. researchers to present new data in an attempt to convince lawmakers that properly regulated IV-B stem cell research was a reliable scientific process with much promise. Benvenisty's research team found that genetically manipulated human blastocyst stem cells have a lower chance of being rejected by the body than other cells. These discoveries give hope that treatment using IV-B stem cell technology is possible in humans.

Dr. Michel Ravel, a professor in the department of molecular genetics at the Weizmann Institute of Science, chaired Israel's Bioethics Committee of the National Committee of Science that wrote the guidelines for Israel's regulations on IV-B research. "Jewish law has a strong tendency towards saving lives," said Ravel. "Therefore, it was easier than in many countries that are under Christian influence to accept the ethical value of the guidelines."[39]

Czech Republic

The Czech Republic is a small country with only a few IV-B stem cell research teams. These teams are motivated by E.U. projects directed by the U.S. and U.K. As a result, biologist Petr Dvorak and his team have stabilized seven new lines of IV-B stem cells that are safer for patients and easier for researchers to use.

Since these lines derived at the Laboratory of Molecular Medicine in Brno were created after August 2001, they are off-limits to scientists using U.S. federal funds for research.

As a part of the Czech Centre for Cell Therapy and Tissue Repair in Prague, Czech researchers are encouraged to develop protocols and strategies for neurodifferentiation of human blastocyst stem cells. This research team, headed by neurobiologist Professor Eva Syková, plans to implant blastocystic stem cells into animals having pathological dysfunction or an injury to the brain or spine. The cells will be marked by nanoparticles traceable using Nuclear Magnetic Resonance.

The Czech Republic has no government funding earmarked exclusively for stem cell research. Researchers have to compete for funding by submitting bids to the Grant Agency of the Czech Republic, the Ministry of Health, or other funding bodies to be reviewed by the system. Once the research project obtains approval from the Bioethical Commission, a registry of eligible stem cells is held at the Ministry of Education. In July 2006 the Czech government adopted legislation similar to the U.K. model: therapeutic cloning (SCNT) is allowed, but reproductive cloning (ANT) is banned.

Turkey

Dr. Necati Findikli of Istanbul Memorial Hospital reported the creation of IV-B stem cell lines in Turkey in 2005. Turkey has no specific guidelines enforced by legal or governmental institutions for IV-B stem cell research.

India

India made the news in the international field of research

when an eye-care and research institute called LV Prasad Eye Institute reported using adult stem cells in the treatment of human eye diseases that were considered untreatable before. India has been able to achieve remarkable progress in this field for two reasons:

- because religious and governmental barriers were not a problem. India's Medical Termination of Pregnancy Act allows termination of pregnancy up to 20 weeks after conception. The Hindu religion does not consider it immoral to conduct research using IV-B stem cells because this research has great potential to alleviate human suffering; therefore, it cannot be considered unethical, and

- because India has a large pool of scientific talent, pharmaceutical and biotechnological companies, and a mature information technology industry.

India was on the verge of becoming known as a biotech powerhouse when its government put the brakes on research that was disorganized and unsafe. After four years of consultations, experts from the Indian Council of Medical Research (ICMR) and the department of biotechnology (DBT) have finalized guidelines that will regulate stem cell research in India. Those guidelines are:

- Genetic engineering or reproductive cloning (ANT) is not allowed.

- The identity of the donor and the recipient will be kept confidential.

- Genetic material (ova and sperm) may not be passed from parents to children.

156

- *In vitro* culture beyond 14 days is not allowed.

- Transfer of human blastocysts into a human or animal uterus after *in vitro* manipulation at any stage of development is not allowed.

- All new stem lines created in India and all imported cell lines must be registered with National Apex Committee for Stem Cell Research and Therapy (NAC-SCRT) and Institutional Committee for Stem Cell Research and Therapy (IC-SCRT)

- Donor consent is mandatory.

- All cord blood banks will be registered with the Drug Controller General of India (DCGI).

- Research using fetal stem cells and placenta will still be permitted, but an abortion may not be sought with intent to donate fetal tissue in return for possible financial or therapeutic benefits.

There are about fifteen institutions in India working on stem cell projects, but those most predominant are:

- Asian Heart Institute and Research Center in Delhi

- Indian Institute of Science in Bangalore

- Maulana Azad Medical College in Delhi

- National Center for Cell Science in Pune

- Ruby Hall Medical Research Center in Pune

- National Centre for Biological Sciences/ Tata Institute of Fundamental Research in Bangalore

- Reliance Life Sciences in Mumbai

Iran

With the approval of Ayatollah Seyed Ali Khamenei, Iran's supreme religious leader, Iranian scientists developed IV-B stem cell lines in 2003. Adult stem cell research is also being conducted in Saudi Arabia and Malaysia.

Asian Countries

Asia is diverse in terms of culture and religion, but overall there is a positive view towards scientific research and medical technology. Most Asians see the value of embryonic stem cell research and its potential to save life. Asia has fewer governmental and religious restrictions regarding protocol for human stem cell research. China, India, Japan, Korea, Singapore, Taiwan, Thailand, and Vietnam do have regulations and some restriction on reproductive cloning. These countries see stem cell research as a way to get ahead in biotechnology.

Asian countries are far from leading the way in stem cells, but they are not about to give up. Susan Lim is the chairman of Stem Cell Technologies, a Singapore startup focusing on ways to extract adult stem cells from fat tissue. Lim said, "I don't think any one country can monopolize stem cell research."[40] She is right; the entire planet will benefit from the technologies and pharmaceuticals developed from stem cell research, regardless of where the research is conducted.

Singapore

Who would have thought that a small island state only forty years old would be the location for one of the best bioresearch centers in the world? That's what happened in July 2000 when Alan Colman, a British scientist who was part of the team that cloned

Dolly the sheep, incorporated his biomedical research company, ES Cell International, in Singapore.

Singapore—a tiny country at the southern tip of the Malay Peninsula—has a diverse population that includes Muslim, Hindu, and Buddhist communities. With only 15 percent of the nation being Christian, and the government fully funding highly regulated IV-B stem cell research, Singapore researchers are able to focus on their science without all the nuances they would have to work around in the U.S. As a result, ES Cell International has been able to commercially produce four lines of IV-B stem cells made in accordance with clinical standards that meet American NIH regulations.

In addition to the $2.94 billion raised by the private sector, the Singapore government, having no national debt, has been able to invest an estimated $949 million on biotechnology since 2000. Another $925 million is slated for release over the next five years. Compare that to the $27 billion that the National Institutes of Health in the U.S. invests annually in biomedical research and it may not seem like much; however, it is enough to entice many top U.S. researchers to move their families or lend their talents to an Asian country no larger than the city of San Diego. Those on the advisory board to Singapore's Biomedical Research Council include:

- David Baltimore of Caltech.

- La Jolla-based scientist John Reed of the Burnham Institute for Medical Research.

- Sydney Brenner of the Salk Institute for Biological Studies.

- Richard Lerner of the Scripps Research Institute.

About $370 million of the Singapore government's biomedical contribution was used to build Biopolis, a massive nine-building, 2.4-million square-foot complex for research and biotechnology. Workers spend long hours on their projects and are addtionally compensated by a government-funded childcare center, dry cleaner, hair salon, supermarket, bars, and even a convenience store on site. As a result, more than 10,000 jobs have been created.

Research conducted at the Biopolis will complement efforts in the United States by working globally with greats such as:

- Stuart Weissman, a pioneer in IV-B stem cell research at Stanford.

- Roger Pedersen, a former researcher at UC San Francisco, who left the United States for England soon after President Bush restricted federal funding of research that uses blastocystic stem cells.

- Blastocystic stem cell researcher Bing Lim from Harvard Medical School.

- University of California San Diego's former medical school dean, Edward Holmes, and his wife, Judith Swain, a cellular cardiologist. The couple leads Singapore's effort to bring medical discoveries into therapies that can be used on patients.

- Dr. Sydney Brenner, a Nobel laureate and professor at the Salk Institute in La Jolla.

- Neal Copeland and Nancy Jenkins, top blastocystic stem cell researchers from the NIH's National Cancer Institute, are working with Lane at the Institute for Cellular and Molecular

Biology. The married couple left the NIH because of the restriction on U.S. funding in scientific research.

• Sai Kiang Lim from State University of New York, Buffalo.

The Singapore government is not only importing talent, it is also drawing students by offering them entry into an 8-year, all-expenses-paid education program. In 2007, Duke University plans to open the first U.S.-style Graduate Medical University in Asia based on Duke's curriculum with faculty also supplied by Duke. Educators Edison Liu, former director of clinical sciences at the U.S. National Cancer Institute, and Massachusetts Institute of Technology's Jackie Ying will be spending much of their time in Singapore.

Since Biopolis opened in 2001, Abbott Laboratories and Novartis have invested millions of dollars in research and drug production facilities in Singapore. Other drug, biotech, and healthcare companies such as Roche, GlaxoSmith Klein, NovoNordisk, and even Carlsbad-based Invitrogen, are investing in the Singapore venture. Johns Hopkins University has set up a stem cell lab in Singapore.

China

China is one of the Asian countries that have been recruiting scientists from top universities in the U.S. to operate research centers on the mainland. China has made tremendous advances in research and treatments derived from all types of stem cells. China has a permissive stance on IV-B stem cell research and SCNT or therapeutic cloning. Some critics see China's approach to oversight and ethics in some labs as lax due to their use of stem cells drawn from fetuses aborted in the second trimester.

RIGHT TO RECOVER—*Yvonne Perry*

Stem Cells China Limited has built partnerships with several leading hospitals across China. The highest professionalism is practiced in research labs, during surgery and after care/ rehabilitation in all the medical centers affiliated with Stem Cells China Limited. One lab is attempting to use stem cells to treat amyotrophic lateral sclerosis (ALS), or Lou Gehrig's disease. Stem Cells China Limited created a service called China Stem Cells, which is a company dedicated to offering the latest news, information, and facts about stem cell research around the globe and medical treatments in China.

Japan

Japanese author, Dr. Kyoko Hayashida, says that Japanese researchers have grown new heart valves in rabbits using cells from the animals' own tissue.

The Institute for Frontier Medical Sciences, Kyoto University was established in 1998 with a goal of learning to use tissues and organs as regeneration tools in future medicine. The Institute has an adjunct facility known as Stem Cell Research Center, which has three laboratories: Laboratory of Embryonic Stem Cell Research (Assoc. Prof. Hirofumi Suemori), Laboratory of Stem Cell Differentiation (Assoc. Prof. Jun Yamashita), and Laboratory of Stem Cell Engineering (Assoc. Prof. Takashi Tada).

Laboratory of Embryonic Stem Cell Research establishes and characterizes human IV-B stem cell lines from material donated with informed consent. These lines are distributed to nationally approved laboratories and used for instruction on culture techniques and to analyze the mechanisms of cell differentiation. The Laboratory of Stem Cell Differentiation studies and learns to control cell differentiation. Laboratory of Stem Cell Engineering in is charge of the engineering of functional tissues from stem cells.

The RIKEN Center for Developmental Biology (CDB) is a large natural sciences research institute in Kobe, Japan. Founded in 1917, the RIKEN Center now has approximately 3000 scientists on seven campuses across Japan, the main one in Wako, just outside Tokyo. Research at the RIKEN Center is funded by the Japanese government with an annual budget of 88 billion yen—equivalent to 760 million U.S. dollars.

With 31 different laboratories, RIKEN CDB conducts research in the field of developmental biology including embryology, developmental cell biology, neural developmental biology, stem cell and tissue regeneration research, and evolutional biology.

Yoshiki Sasai and the team at RIKEN CDB developed a new system to stimulate IV-B stem cells to differentiate into neuron cells in a culture dish. By coating the cells with human amniotic membrane, the precursor stem cells gave rise to diverse types of neurons located in multiple regions of the brain. The lab-generated neuron cells responded to external stimuli in a manner similar to neural precursor cells developing within an actual brain of a mouse or human embryo. The team plans to determine whether these cells can replicate therapeutic activity in animal models of Parkinson's disease. Sasai's work is reported in the *Proceedings of the National Academy of Sciences.*

South Korea

Over the past two years Seoul has dished out a total of $27 million in public money for stem cell research. In spite of being disgraced by the scientific misconduct of cloning expert Dr. Woo Suk Hwang, South Koreans continued to support him and his work. Upon hearing of the falsifying of his scientific reports, message boards were bombarded with those voicing their support for the renowned scientist. His articles published in *Science* were withdrawn when the Seoul National University (SNU) proved that Woo-Suk's work contained fabricated data and altered photos.

The scandal did not stop research efforts by veterinarian Woo-suk Hwang. After he resigned from SNU, he collected private funding to set up a new laboratory. His former staff was willing to continue working with him. However, the Health Ministry revoked his license, which means he will not have access to eggs necessary for his research. That's when South Korean women rallied and began offering to donate their eggs for Hwang's IV-B research efforts.

Hwang is currently facing trial for the misappropriation of state and private funds worth an estimated 2.8 billion won (around 2.5 million euros) and for buying the eggs needed for his experiments, a practice forbidden by the country's bioethics law.

Japan is especially concerned with patents that will protect intellectual property (IP) created at universities, research institutions, and biological or life-science industries and to prevent dangerous exploitation of human material as a source of profit. Unlike individual-minded materialist Western countries, these community-oriented countries aim to create and contribute new knowledge internationally and promote a safe, high-quality life for all. Abiding by a policy that egg and sperm donors must give informed consent to participate in the research, some Asian countries will not use cell lines created by Professor Woo Suk Hwang's team. Their scientific journals refuse to publish the results of any unethical research. Singaporean research company hESCell International plans to share data and cell lines with international researchers in Australia, the United Kingdom, Israel, Germany, Sweden, the Netherlands, Japan, Canada, France, Finland, and the United States.

Three major centers for stem cell research are: MizMedi Hospital – Seoul National University, Pochon CHA University, and Maria Biotech Co. Ltd.– Maria Infertility Hospital Medical Institute all located in Seoul, Korea.

African Countries

Linked to the University of Stellenbosch, a privately owned company in South Africa named Lazaron Biotechnologies set up the first stem cell bank in South Africa. The bank, which opened in 2005, harvests and cryogenically stores cord blood for research and treatment of a range of diseases. Lazaron Biotechnologies also has an interest in animal biology. In addition to its Human Stem Cell Bank, its Regenerative Cell Technology Division, and Future Regenerative Treatment Facilities, the company also conducts research in its Animal Bio-Cell Division. Larazon holds an exclusive license for all the technologies that come from animal and human stem cell research at the biotechnology laboratories in the Department of Animal Sciences of the University of Stellenbosch.

Today there are three cord blood banks in South Africa.

Egypt

In October 2005, scientists began conducting stem cell research in Egypt through a private Egyptian IVF Center in Cairo. The research began using stem cells from umbilical cord blood. Clinical director Gamal Serour would like to use surplus IV-Bs from consenting couples, but Egypt, like most deeply conservative and religious Muslim countries, is divided on the moral issue of blastocystic stem cell research. Some Islamic experts on Sharia (Islamic law) believe the soul enters an embryo on the 120th day of the pregnancy and gains its moral status or rights as a person. Other Islamic scholars say the soul enters an embryo on the 40th day after conception. But others say it is immoral, even infanticide, to destroy embryos at any stage.

Obviously, Hamdy el-Sayed, the Muslim president of the Egyptian Medical Syndicate, did not know the difference between fertilization and conception when he said, "It's (an *in vitro* blastocyst) already a human life at conception." *In vitro* fertilized eggs that are not implanted are not at the conception stage, which must occur within the uterus.

According to Dr. Muzammil Siddiqi, chairman of the Islamic Law Council of North America, the Sharia makes a distinction between potential life and actual life. "Although life begins at conception in the womb, an embryo formed by artificial fertilization is not in its natural environment.... If it is not placed in the womb it will not survive and it will not become a human being." Dr. Siddiqi believes stem cells should be derived only from therapeutic cloning or from excess frozen IV-Bs.

According to Thomas Eich, a researcher on Islamic bioethics at Bochum University in Germany, there are no Egyptian laws regarding IV-B stem cells. Dr. Serour, the Director at International Islamic Center for Population Studies and Research in Cairo, argues that IV-B stem cells should be used for research to benefit human beings rather than allowing them to perish.

The Egyptian Medical Syndicate, a governing body, forbids the use of any blastocysts for experimentation. In 2003, a scholar in Cairo comparing therapeutic cloning of blastocysts to the accepted practice of donating cells, tissues, or organs for transplants, issued an Islamic religious ruling stating that SCNT is to be considered lawful. The Academy of Scientific Research and Technology in Egypt support both IV-B stem cell research and therapeutic cloning.

Fear owns no particular denomination or sect, but seems to be common in most religions. According to Zaghloul el-Naggar, an Egyptian expert on Islam and science, Muslim officials are concerned that therapeutic cloning could lead to abuses such as the cloning and murder of babies to supply organs or spare parts for patients, or people selling or using surplus *in vitro* fertilized eggs without consent of the parents. Dr. Ragaa Mansour, scientific director and program manager of the Egyptian IVF Center, says, "How can we ban anything just because it can be misused? We should regulate and prevent misuse of technology [and] encourage research in the right direction."

So far, the Egyptian government doesn't appear to be taking any rash actions. "It's important for the government to support it, and I do encourage stem cell research," says Salah Labib, director general of the Ministry of Health and Population's Specialized Medical Committee, a governmental arm responsible for funding well-established treatments. Dr. Labib says he would be open to financing future stem cell therapies, provided they are safer, easier, and cheaper than some of the treatments the government is financing now. "But I think every research should ... be ethically evaluated first," he says.

Australia

ES Cell International's corporate headquarters are housed within a leading Australian Medical Research Precinct. ES Cell is a regenerative medicine company focusing on developing therapeutic products from blastocyst stem cells. Incorporated in 2000, the company funds research with four collaborating research centers: The Monash Institute of Reproduction and Development (Australia), the National University of Singapore (Singapore), Hadassah Medical Organization (Israel), and the Hubrecht Laboratory (the Netherlands).

In 2002, ES Cell International in Australia held six of the 22 IV-B stem cell lines having met the requirements set forth by the Bush administration in 2001. These were listed on the NIH Stem Cell Registry. ES Cell International and the NIH signed the federal government's first international agreement involving the distribution of human stem cell lines. The Memorandum of Understanding (MOU) for research allowed for accessibility to those six cell lines in compliance with the NIH guidelines for the transfer of research materials to individual laboratories. The NIH will retain ownership to any new intellectual property that might arise from research in this area. ES Cell International will receive a fee to cover its handling and distribution expenses in supplying these cell lines and will retain commercial rights to its materials.

Australia's Parliament passed its first laws on stem cell research in 2002, allowing scientists to extract stem cells from IV-Bs but preventing any type of cell cloning. In December 2006, despite opposition from conservative Prime Minister John Howard and other party leaders, Australia's parliament lifted a ban on SCNT cloning for stem cell research. The law will come into effect after health and science authorities draft guidelines for egg donation and research licenses.

Former Health Minister Kay Patterson, the senator who drafted the bill, said, "This work's being done in Sweden, England, the United States, in Japan . . . and I didn't see how we could accept any treatment derived from this in the future if we didn't allow the research here in Australia."

There are over 70,000 IV-Bs in Australia alone and many of them are slated for destruction. Using them for scientific research utilizes a resource that would otherwise be wasted. How appropriate that the 5th Annual Meeting of the International Society for Stem Cell Research was held June 17–21, 2007, at the Cairns Convention Centre in Cairns, Australia.

Canada

The Canadian Institutes of Health Research (CIHR) is the major federal agency responsible for funding health research in Canada. The CIHR has set guidelines regarding the use of stem cells for public funding. These guidelines do not affect private funding nor do they have legal implications. Here is a brief outline of some of the CIHR guidelines:

- Must use leftover *in vitro* blastocysts created to help couples conceive. Blastocysts should not be created solely for research purposes.

- The couples must give informed consent for these cells to be used in research. This consent must be renewed at the time of the actual research so donors have a second opportunity to change their minds.

- The cells must not be more than 14 days old.

- Cloning human bodies is not allowed.

- Combining non-human stem cells with human cells is not allowed.

- Donors are not allowed to receive monetary payment for the donation or creation of reproductive material.

- Research on stem cell lines created outside of Canada will only be permitted if the lines were created in accordance with CIHR's guidelines.

Canada's policy seems on the mark when it comes to being ethical and allowing research on IV-B stem cells to flourish.

A Calgary-based company, Stem Cell Therapeutics has approved two drugs: Human chorionic gonadotropin (hCG) and Erythropoietin (EPO) to stimulate stem cell activity in the brain of patients who have had a stroke. It is hoped that this therapy called NTxTM-265 will provide benefit through the replacement of brain cells that were lost or damaged by the stroke. Clinical trials are beginning to investigate the safety and efficacy of NTxTM-265 in humans.

South American Countries

Practical use of stem cells is not a dream in the distant future. Two kidney dialysis patients from Argentina received the world's first tissue-engineered blood vessels fashioned from their own skin and vein tissue.

In 2004, Amit Patel and a team from University of Pittsburg School of Medicine conducted a trial in South America using adult stem cells. The study included 20 patients, but only half received stem cell therapy during by-pass surgery for heart failure. Stem cells harvested from the patient's own bone marrow were injected into the heart where there was evidence of damaged muscle. The results show that those who had the injections were able to pump more blood than those who had surgery alone. It is hoped that stem cells are able to help regenerate the heart muscle and stimulate the formation of new blood vessels. In January 2005, Patel injected bone marrow stem cells into cardiac tissue of congestive heart failure patients who were not having surgery. Six months later, there was marked improvement similar to the study mentioned above.

In Brazil, forty-one stem cell projects conducted in 2005 and 2006 shared nearly $5 million in funding from the Brazilian Government. Three of the projects used IV-B stem cells alone, four used both adult and blastocystic cells, and 34 used adult cells alone. Brazil's policies on IV-B stem cells permits research only on remaining fertilized eggs no longer needed for reproduction. Brazil is a Catholic country and does not allow SCNT cloning at all.

Chapter Nine

PUBLIC OPINION ABOUT STEM CELL RESEARCH

On July 17, 2006 the Senate passed H.R. 810 the Stem Cell Research Enhancement Act of 2005 in a vote of 63 to 37. That's only four votes short of the needed tally to override a presidential veto. With the passage of this bill, many people had their hopes raised that research utilizing stem cells from frozen IV-Bs would be allowed and that a cure might be found for those who suffer with spinal cord injury, Alzheimer's, diabetes and other serious illnesses. On July 19, President Bush dashed their hopes with a veto that the House was unable to override.

I really don't like to use a lot of statistics because most people find them boring. However, I need reliable data to support my findings—otherwise all you have is my opinion and I've already harped about making decisions based upon opinion rather than facts.

I realize that poll results can be tainted by who is asking the questions. For example, if your minister or priest asked you if you support "embryonic" stem cell research, you might fear his rejection enough to say "no". On the other hand, if you were answering a survey in which you were allowed to remain anonymous, you might be inclined to say "yes". Additionally, opinions vary upon how poll questions are worded. For example, if a pro-life organization were to poll people, they might use emotional language to gain support for their cause by asking the question: "Do you believe a live human embryo should be destroyed to advance scientific research?" If a major foundation supporting stem cell research were to poll the same people, they might use technical or scientific data to bring about support for their cause: "Do you believe stem cells leftover from *in vitro* procedures should be used to find life-saving cures for diseases or injuries?"

Even though there is a margin for error, polls are a reasonable method for showing current patterns and belief systems in a wide range of people. In some places in this chapter, I averaged the data whenever there was a wide variation of percentages on surveys conducted near the same time. The statistics were gathered from several nationwide surveys: Harris Interactive®, Newsweek, ABCNEWS/Beliefnet, Genetics and Public Policy Center (GPPC) and the Coalition for the Advancement of Medical Research (CAMR).

Let's take a look at the issues. I say issues (plural) because we are looking at two factors: *in vitro* blastocyst stem cell research in general and the funding of such by using taxpayer dollars. I'll begin by reviewing how Americans personally feel about blastocyst stem cell research in general.

Stem Cell Research in General

After an announcement was made that a way had been found to harvest stem cells without harming the blastocyst, Newsweek interviewed 1,002 adults aged 18 and older on August 24 and 25,

2006 to see what influence this information had on the American public. The results of that 2006 poll show that approximately 65 percent of American voters favor IV-B research in general and 36 percent oppose it.[41] The statistics hadn't changed much from Newsweek's 2001 poll which showed approximately 66 percent in favor. However, a poll conducted by CAMR found 72 percent of Americans in favor of advancing IV-B stem cell research. ABC News/Washington Post Poll conducted a poll on January 16-19, 2007 asked respondents, "Do you support or oppose embryonic stem cell research?" Sixty-one percent said they supported, 31 percent opposed, and 8 percent were unsure.[42]

From a combination and average of all the polls I've researched, there is an approximate 7:1 ratio in favor of IV-B research. Congressman Jim Langevin of Rhode Island said, "I'm willing to bet those in the remaining percentage haven't been educated on the issues." I agree, which is precisely why I wrote this book. Educating the public allows people to make informed decisions.

Federal Funding for Research

About half the survey respondents mentioned above say that the federal government should fund IV-B research; 40 percent oppose it; the others were undecided. Since these results are consistent with the Newsweek Poll conducted in October 2004 during the presidential campaign, this data shows that the same number of voters support funding for IV-B research regardless of whether they are told an embryo is destroyed in the process.

Why do people favor federal funding for IV-B research? Of the 48 percent who support federal funding more than three-fourths (77%) of them say they do so because they support scientific progress in general. Less than one-fourth (21%) of them support it because they have or know someone who has a medical condition that might be helped by the research. Of the 36 percent of the population that opposes federal funding for the research 49 percent say it would not be a good use of public money. Forty-six percent of them say it conflicts with their religious or moral values. If my math is correct (46% of the 36% opposed) and the statistics are accurate, funding for IV-B research conflicts with the religious or moral values of only 16.6 percent of Americans.

Why has our president and senate chosen to cater to a minority of voices who oppose federal funding for blastocystic stem cell research when almost 65 percent of our citizens clearly support it? Could it be ignorance? Dan Bloodworth told me that he is sure that if he had as much as fifteen minutes with George W. Bush accompanied by Senator Frist, he could change the president's mind. After Dan sat with Senator Frist and shared his Biblical support for IV-B technology, the former doctor turned politician said, "I've read that book (the Bible) front to back more than one time, Brother Dan, but I would never have put together what you have just shown me." He agreed IV-B stem cell research must be a gift from God.

President Bush still believes that using IV-B stem cells for any research purpose raises serious ethical questions. His stance may help put a Democrat in the Oval Office in 2008. By the way, in the same 2006 Newsweek Poll mentioned above, only 31 percent of respondents approve of the way the president is handling the issue of federally funded stem cell research, while 52 percent disapprove. Sixty-five percent of the respondents of the poll say they are dissatisfied with the general way things are going in the United States; only 28 percent are satisfied.

RIGHT TO RECOVER—*Yvonne Perry*

Poll Demographics

Next, let's look at the demographics obtained through polls.

Religion

According to ABCNEWS/Beliefnet poll approximately three in ten adults oppose stem cell research in general due to their religious beliefs. This shows the amount of power religious leaders have to sway their congregations.

Attitudes toward IV-B research vary depending on denomination and how dedicated the individual is to her or his religious practice. "Born-again" Christians who attend religious services every week are more likely to oppose IV-B research. Evangelical white Protestants are a conservative, anti-abortion group of religious people largely supportive of the Bush administration. About as many evangelical white Protestants (50%) as white Catholics (54%) are in favor of IV-B research while seventy percent of white non-evangelical Protestants support it. Strangely, sixty percent of the Catholic population favors its federal funding as a matter of policy. This suggests that even within these groups there is not a lot of opposition to IV-B research. In fact, many Catholics and Jesuits are taking a more liberal view of religion and the world. The mainstream Catholic Church in America is not in opposition to blastocyst stem cell research. Catholics for a Free Choice is a group that has pulled away from the official Papal viewpoint of Rome and joined together with the majority of U.S. Catholics who support IV-B stem cell research.

Catholic opposition to the research comes mainly from its leadership and not its laity. Religious leaders were not moved by the discovery that a method had been found to use a single stem cell to produce additional stem cell lines without bothering the rest of the cells in the blastocyst. Richard Doerflinger, Pro-life Activities Deputy Director at the U.S. Conference of Catholic Bishops still believes an IV-B clump of cells is equal to a human life. He says he cannot support the discovery because IV-B stem cells were destroyed in the research process that led to the new discovery. He asked his followers, "Why do we need embryonic stem cells at all? ...even the latest studies show disappointing results...."[43]

Where is the logic or compassion in Doerflinger's statement? The IV-Bs leftover from fertility attempts will be thrown away if they are not used for research. Then, why not let the leftovers serve as research material rather than filler for the trash can? The only way to keep from destroying the leftover IV-B stem cells is to implant all the blastocysts or do away with *in vitro* fertilization all together. And in Italy that is exactly what the Vatican would like to see happen.

Italy's IVF law says a woman cannot utilize IVF unless she's married. She can't use donated eggs or sperm so that does away with surrogacy. To them, surrogacy is equal to a married man or woman having sex with another man or woman to whom they are not married. Only three eggs can be fertilized at a time and all three blastocysts have to be implanted into the womb. That means a woman could conceive multiple pregnancies simultaneously. Worse yet, the triplets may have a disease or be deformed. A doctor who violates any part of the IVF law can be imprisoned for up to three years. In 2005, Italians held a referendum on whether to change the law on fertility treatments and stem cell research. Those efforts failed because Catholic bishops, with the support of Pope Benedict XVI, persuaded registered voters to stay away from the polls. Talk about religious control and loss of free will—that tops it all. The scientists who are trying to find cures are not interested in creating Frankensteins. Religious and political leaders are the monsters we need to worry about!

It's not right to deny anyone the privilege of being able to have children through *in vitro* assistance. I don't think anyone wants to lose the remarkable IVF procedure in the U.S, but if we don't open our eyes and start taking action to put a stop to the control religion and government has over us, we will soon be in no better shape than Italy.

If U.S. Catholics are pro-life, why would their leaders oppose a valuable scientific discovery that indicates it has the potential to save or improve life? Has not one Catholic or pro-life couple ever used *in vitro* technology to conceive a child in the U.S.? What about their leftover blastocyst cells? Are they all adopted by surrogate parents? I seriously doubt it. There are only three choices remaining: do like Italy and implant all the blastocysts, pay to have the cells preserved (although their shelf life is not eternal), or throw them away. A fourth and better choice is to let them be used for research in hopes of bringing about treatment for disease and injury.

When it comes to ideology the breakdown across America shows 44 percent of Conservatives, 63 percent of Moderates and 76 percent of Liberals support IV-B research. The highest opposition to stem cell research is among the one in five Americans who think abortion should be illegal in all cases. Those people must not realize there is a huge difference between abortion and IV-B stem cell research. Pro-stem cell advocates must separate the false assumption of stem cell science with abortion issues promoted by the opposition. They are not the same—not even close.

Race

Sixty percent of the Caucasian population approves IV-B

research while only forty-eight percent of the Black community approves it. I found this surprising since African-Americans are the most solidly Democratic group in the nation. As you will see later in this chapter, Democrats are more supportive of IV-B research than are Republicans. Lower support was shown among non-English speaking Hispanics.

Demographic factors such as age, income or gender showed little variation in views. Key factors are religion, education levels, and politics.

Education

Education does seem to be a factor in those who support funding for IV-B research. Sixty-four percent of respondents who are college graduates support federal funding while 46 percent of those with a high school education or less oppose funding. Those who have a better understanding of the issues also support funding for the research. Of the 65 percent who support the research in general, 49 percent of them say they understand IV-B research and *in vitro* fertilization issues somewhat well, while 26 percent say they understand it very well, and 24 percent say they don't understand the issue at all.

A poll in 2001 showed that only 68 percent of the population had seen, heard or read about the debate on whether to allow stem cell research. In 2004, eighty-three percent at least knew something about the issue. In the 2001 poll, 32 percent believed that "allowing any medical research using stem cells from human embryos should be forbidden because it is unethical and immoral." That number had decreased to 15 percent by 2004. One question the survey asked was, "Do you believe that using stem cells from human embryos for research comes too close to allowing scientists play God?" In 2001, forty percent said yes. In 2004, only nineteen percent still held that belief.

Politics

Another demographic consideration noted by the polls is that of political persuasion. Remember that within a group of people labeled the same, there is a wide variety of personal opinion and belief not consistent with that of the affiliated party. While not all Republicans or Democrats are either for or against blastocystic stem cell research and its funding, we are looking at the consensus of the majority in this context.

Republicans

Republicans are less likely than Democrats to approve of IV-B research in general. Polls conducted in 2004 revealed that sixty percent of Republicans and eighty percent of Democrats believe IV-B research should be allowed. However, when it comes to spending taxpayer dollars to fund the research, sixty percent of Democrats think Bush should change his position on federal funding for IV-B research, while only 36 percent of Republicans say he should.

Senator Bill Frist

One influential person of that thirty-six percent is former Republican Senator Bill Frist. As a supporter of IV-B research, Dr. Frist believes the presidents' policy regarding the Congress-approved H.R. 810, the Stem Cell Research Enhancement Act of 2005, should be modified. Dr. Frist is an avowed Christian. His support for IV-B research seemed contradictory to some, but the man knows what he's talking about. He is a heart-lung transplant

surgeon who understands biology and can easily see the benefits
this technology could bring to the healthcare field. On July 28,
2005, he defended his position by saying:

> *I am pro-life; I believe human life begins at conception. I
> also believe that embryonic stem cell research should be encouraged
> and supported. An embryo is nascent human life. This position is
> consistent with my faith. But, to me, it isn't just a matter of faith.
> It's a fact of science. The government should pay for research only
> on those embryos that would be discarded otherwise. ...Cure today
> may be just a theory, a hope, a dream, but the promise is powerful
> enough that I believe this research deserves our increased energy and
> focus. Embryonic stem cell research must be supported. It's time for
> a modified policy - the right policy for this moment in time.[44]*

Frist says that life begins at conception. Obviously, he knows
that fertilization and conception are separate events. Frist also
mentioned President Bush's announcement in 2001 that authorized
the release of 78 stem cell lines that would be eligible for federal
money. At the time of Frist's speech there were only 22 eligible
lines. The others had been developed using animal feeder layers of
cells and are therefore not usable for research seeking to develop
treatments for humans.

The FDA ruled that those cell lines created with animal feeders
be excluded from NIH–sponsored research. As of the writing of
this book, there were only 19 lines available and 12 of them are still
being tested for usability. Even if these lines meet Bush-approved
criterion, it does not mean they will meet the strict ethical standards
enforced by many universities. Researchers need to be able to utilize
cell lines created without animal feeder layers using the newest and
best technologies, which have been discovered since August of

2001. The technology used for harvesting blastocyst stem cells has improved greatly in the past six years. The newer cells renew more quickly for reproducibility and would include diversity in race and genetic types.

Ron Reagan

The younger son of the late Republican President Reagan, Ron Reagan, spoke at the 2004 Democratic National Convention in Boston in favor of stem cell research. He believes it is important to the country and the world that we talk about blastocystic stem cell research, especially since President Bush does not support the research and most Democrats do.

Republican President Bush has not opposed all stem cell research—he allows research on the cell lines created before August 9, 2001—the tainted ones already on death-by-trash-can row. The arbitrary nature of the Bush policy shows that he is not convinced that embryos are destroyed in the research process or truly concerned about helping people get well. His compromise severely restricted, but did not eliminate blastocystic stem cell research. The U.S. provided funding of $24.8 million for human blastocyst stem cell research in 2003. In contrast, the Bush Administration allotted $190.7 million for adult stem cells, including those from cord blood, placenta, and bone marrow.

President Bush can be characterized as "ultra right wing" but that is not the position of the majority of people in this nation. A significant number of Republican voters do not feel the same way about IV-B research as do the national party leaders. An average of all polls show that seventy percent of American voters approve of IV-B research in general and about fifty percent believe the federal government should fund the research; forty percent oppose it and the other ten percent are undecided. A poll by Genetics and Public Policy Center showed that fifty-nine percent of people want more lenient federal research policies than currently exist. From the data I have collected, I have come to the understanding that Americans do value human blastocysts, but they also understand the tremendous benefits of IV-B research. They would rather give science a chance to explore the untapped curative potential than defend a clump of cells about to be destroyed in a laboratory.

What type of leader would ignore the wishes of seventy-two percent of his constituents and the advice of leading experts in this scientific field of study? The same type of person who would send troops into a war without the consent of Congress; the same type of person who did not immediately or sufficiently respond to the needs of residents in areas devastated by Hurricane Katrina; the same type of person who just weeks after terrorist attacks on September 11, 2001 would rapidly enact the USA Patriot Act without giving Congress time to read through its 342 pages or debate its contents; the same man who would reauthorize the USA Patriot Act in March 2006 saying he did not feel obliged to obey requirements that he inform Congress about how the FBI was using the act's expanded police powers; the same man who would veto a bill that had passed through Congress with sixty-seven percent of the vote. Obviously, this same man does not want to be held accountable for his actions or have his unauthorized power contested. And, people believe what he has to say about blastocyst stem cells? Strange, isn't it?

Democrats

This battle for health and hope will continue to be a topic of heated debate in the next few years. Not only has this fight moved to the states where citizens are taking the issue into their own

hands, it will undoubtedly be a leveraging issue for the Democratic
Party in the 2008 Presidential Election. Looking for issues where
large majorities oppose the tactics of President Bush, IV-B
research must be very attractive. I'm not surprised to note that
eighty percent of Democrats believe that IV-B research should be
allowed. Of course, stem cell research is not the only leveraging
tool the Democrats will use. The U.S. economy, our involvement
in the war in Iraq, and immigration issues will also be used by the
Democratic Party to show how out of step the Republican Party is
with the mainstream.

Let's see how Democratic leaders feel about stem cell
research.

Howard Dean

Former governor of Vermont, Howard Dean, is Chairman
of the Democratic National Committee and the founder of
Democracy for America, a grassroots organization that supports
socially progressive and fiscally responsible political candidates. He
is also a medical doctor and a vocal supporter of stem cell research.
In an article published by Cagle Cartoons, Inc., Dr. Howard Dean
gave an impressive comment about IV-B stem cell research:

*There is no guarantee that stem cell research can produce a cure
for Alzheimer's disease. But stem cells show promise by helping to
prevent or cure chronic and life-shortening diseases such as diabetes,
multiple sclerosis, Parkinson's and various cardiac diseases.*

*Many Republicans continue to link stem cell research to the
abortion debate. Nothing could be further from the truth. Embryonic
stem cells come from embryos which have been created for the purpose
of helping infertile couples have children. In this process, a few*

embryos may be implanted in a woman's uterus, to be born nine months later. A much larger number of embryos will be frozen for future use. The vast majority of these will ultimately be discarded. But, these discarded embryos can produce something good; they can potentially save the life or health of a stranger. Stem cells, the basis of all the cells in our body, can be saved from these embryos, and can become tissue which can potentially replace diseased tissue in human beings who are suffering greatly, as President Reagan did. Or these embryos can be discarded, as they usually are now.

What Mrs. Reagan and other advocates of stem cell research are asking is that the embryos be put to humanitarian and scientific uses, instead of being wasted. Perhaps the research will fail. But, if we do not try, we will never know. President Bush has confined stem cell research to such a few cell lines, which makes most American research meaningless.

Most of the research is now going on in other countries, with a few exceptions in the US, such as wealthy universities that can afford to refuse federal funding. This means that Americans who suffer these diseases will be last in line to get the benefits of this potentially extraordinary research. It also means a generation of American scientists and doctors will fall behind their foreign counterparts in using whatever lifesaving technologies come out of this research.

As a physician, I am embarrassed that America would willingly and deliberately choose to set aside science and the hope it offers. As a Democrat, I say to Nancy Reagan, I'll do whatever I can to help you win this one for the Gipper.[45]

Nancy Pelosi

Representative Nancy Pelosi (D-CA) is the first woman in American history to lead a major party in the U.S. Congress. Beginning in January 2007 as the House Democratic Leader, Representative Pelosi has already made it clear that she will support federal funding for all types of stem cell research. At a Washington, D.C. news conference, Pelosi said:

> *Every family in America is one phone call or one diagnosis away from needing the benefits of stem cell research. The American people have spoken. Seventy-two percent of Americans support ethically based stem cell research. In vetoing this legislation, the President would be saying 'No' to 72 percent of the American people. He would be saying 'No' to so many families across America who are hoping and praying this legislation becomes public policy. He would be saying 'No' to hope.*
>
> *Here we have a special day in the history of our country and this Congress. Important legislation has passed that affects every family in America. And may I say to all of you who have advocated for this; 'Every family in America is in your debt because of your advocacy, your eloquence, and your leadership.' Let's hope your message is not lost on the President of the United States.*
>
> *This research has the biblical power to cure. How can we turn away from that? Let's all pray the President will have a change of heart and a change of mind. But if not, let's work very hard to make sure that Members of Congress represent their constituents and override a presidential veto.*[46]

Representative Pelosi has already confronted Republican leaders regarding continuing to spend money to send more troops to the war in Iraq. I can see her continuing to stir up much needed, eye-opening discussion on issues that have been swept under the rug. Too bad she isn't running for President in 2008. I'd vote for her.

Speaking of voting, here is how your senator voted on H.R. 810 regarding federal funding for IV-B research in July 2006:[47]

Akaka (D-HI), Yea

Alexander (R-TN), Yea

Allard (R-CO), Nay

Allen (R-VA), Nay

Baucus (D-MT), Yea

Bayh (D-IN), Yea

Bennett (R-UT), Yea

Biden (D-DE), Yea

Bingaman (D-NM), Yea

Bond (R-MO), Nay

Boxer (D-CA), Yea

Brownback (R-KS), Nay

Bunning (R-KY), Nay

Burns (R-MT), Nay

Burr (R-NC), Yea

Byrd (D-WV), Yea

Cantwell (D-WA),

Carper (D-DE), Yea

Chafee (R-RI), Yea

Chambliss (R-GA), Nay

Clinton (D-NY), Yea

Coburn (R-OK), Nay

Cochran (R-MS), Yea

Coleman (R-MN), Nay

Collins (R-ME), Yea

Conrad (D-ND), Yea

Inouye (D-HI), Yea

Isakson (R-GA), Nay

Jeffords (I-VT), Yea

Johnson (D-SD), Yea

Kennedy (D-MA), Yea

Kerry (D-MA), Yea

Kohl (D-WI), Yea

Kyl (R-AZ), Nay

Landrieu (D-LA), Yea

Lautenberg (D-NJ), Yea

Leahy (D-VT), Yea

Levin (D-MI), Yea

Lieberman (D-CT), Yea

Lincoln (D-AR), Yea

Lott (R-MS), Yea

Lugar (R-IN), Yea

McCain (R-AZ), Yea

McConnell (R-KY), Nay

Menendez (D-NJ), Yea

Mikulski (D-MD), Yea

Murkowski (R-AK), Yea

Murray (D-WA), Yea

Nelson (D-FL), Yea

Nelson (D-NE), Nay

Obama (D-IL), Yea

Pryor (D-AR), Yea

Cornyn (R-TX), Nay
Craig (R-ID), Nay
Crapo (R-ID), Nay
Dayton (D-MN), Yea
DeMint (R-SC), Nay
DeWine (R-OH), Nay
Dodd (D-CT), Yea
Dole (R-NC), Nay
Domenici (R-NM), Nay
Dorgan (D-ND), Yea
Durbin (D-IL), Yea
Ensign (R-NV), Nay
Enzi (R-WY), Nay
Feingold (D-WI), Yea
Feinstein (D-CA), Yea
Frist (R-TN), Yea
Graham (R-SC), Nay
Grassley (R-IA), Nay
Gregg (R-NH), Yea
Hagel (R-NE), Nay
Harkin (D-IA), Yea
Hatch (R-UT), Yea
Hutchison (R-TX), Yea
Inhofe (R-OK), Nay

Reed (D-RI), Yea
Reid (D-NV), Yea
Roberts (R-KS), Nay
Rockefeller (D-WV), Yea
Salazar (D-CO), Yea
Santorum (R-PA), Nay
Sarbanes (D-MD), Yea
Schumer (D-NY), Yea
Sessions (R-AL), Nay
Shelby (R-AL), Nay
Smith (R-OR), Yea
Snowe (R-ME), Yea
Specter (R-PA), Yea
Stabenow (D-MI), Yea
Stevens (R-AK), Yea
Sununu (R-NH), Nay
Talent (R-MO), Nay
Thomas (R-WY), Nay
Thune (R-SD), Nay
Vitter (R-LA), Nay
Voinovich (R-OH), Nay
Warner (R-VA), Yea
Wyden (D-OR), Yea
Martinez (R-FL), Nay

Centrist Groups

Support for stem cell research is much higher among centrist groups. The Independent Party shows the highest support (83%) for IV-B research. Sixty-three percent of moderates and seventy percent of non-evangelicals are for it. Independents are not held down by partisan ideology and are not influenced as heavily by religion.

Libertarians

Alicia Mattson, Chair of the Libertarian Party of Tennessee, confirmed that stem cell research has not been an issue that the Libertarian Party has discussed or debated. "We've really been focused on ballot access issues," says Mattson. "This issue is similar to the abortion issue—you have Libertarians that are in favor and those that are opposed. When asked about funding for stem cell research she replied, "Libertarians do not support federal funding for hESC research. As with all research, we'd like to see funds raised from the private sector."

Perhaps the Libertarians do not understand how science moves from the lab to the clinic. It takes federal funds and oversight to get anything past the FDA and into the human trial stages.

The Perry Survey

I conducted my own survey during the writing of this book. Between January 22 and February 5, 2007, I polled 88 people with five questions and an opportunity to give a comment. Most of the responders live in the Bible Belt where conservative/fundamental attitudes are elevated. Here are the questions I asked and the tally of the results:

1. How much do you know about blastocyst (also called embryonic) stem cell research?

a. Very little (11.4 %)

b. Only what I've heard/read in the media (59.1%)

C. A lot; I've done some research (29.5%)

2. Some people believe blastocyst stem cell research kills an embryo. Do you:
    a. Agree (21.6 %)
    b. Disagree (78.4 %)

3. Do you believe there is hope that stem cell research may someday provide cures or treatments for disease or injury?
    a. Yes (93.2 %)
    b. No (6.8 %)

4. Should the U.S. government provide funding for research done on blastocyst stem cells?
    a. Yes (76.1%) Notice how the percentages dropped when people were asked to open their wallets!
    b. No (23.9 %)

5. What is your religious affiliation or denomination?
Agnostic/Atheist: 8.7%
Buddhist: 3.5%
Christian/Catholic: 4%
Christian/Protestant: 64.3%
Jewish: 3.5%
None at all: 4%
Pagan/Nature-based: 12%

6. Any other comments?
Note: I corrected spelling and punctuation simply to make the comments clearer, but I have not corrected the responders' grammar or changed any statements made even though some comments given by participants are not supported by scientific facts:
    • A cell without any potential of being a baby, yet the owner is

willing to donate it in order to provide goodness to the already living but perhaps injured is accepted. But, the formation of cell already being a baby, and already living, although willingly donated by the owner, to be killed for the same intention, is not accepted. The God has made all life sacred.

- Adult stem cell research could be funded through the government. It appears to be a more likely candidate for cures in the short term.

- All worldly (or outer) objects are good or bad, dualistic in their nature. The good of blastocyst stem cell research can bring can out weigh the bad that can also be done with it. That would be my prayer.

- Baby Killers!

- Every day humanity wages war upon itself. I find it ludicrous for a government to ban stem cell research on the grounds of morality and yet uphold the death penalty or wage a war.

- Everything is connected. Of course killing a blastocyst kills the embryo it will become, and the baby the embryo will become. The implication is that human (baby) life is the most important value and there are many values with simultaneous importance.

- From what I do know about it, I think it's a great thing and I believe it could cure many illnesses.

- Heard that there has been some research to show that the stem cells are in the amniotic fluid and the placenta. If that can be continued, then the issue of the embryonic stem cell research will not be the only choice. The doctor who reported it on

NPR from a medical magazine is the one doing the research. You might look into it...and he said it would be years before perfected.

- I am for it!!

- I am not against stem cell research but I don't think it should be funded by the government. I also think the underlying moral issue lies with the fertility clinics that allow them to be created in the first place.

- I don't know much about it, but it seems that there are options to do the research without having to use an embryo; however, if the embryos are from abortions (which are still legal), it does seem like one way to have something "good" come from that situation. However, I also think that growing organs and other research seems to show similar promise in finding cures for many diseases. So overall, I support the research, but also support viable alternatives.

- I feel research is important. But to take a life to do so, just to be able to sustain another life isn't the answer. This will create more "abortions on demand"...

- I find it extremely hypocritical for someone to be so cavalier about sending adult men and women to be killed in war, but yet can't see the benefits to humankind from Stem cell research...what's wrong with this picture? Greed...

- I had trouble with your question #2. Whether or not I believe it "kills an embryo" is sort of beside the point. I think the question is, am I OK with embryonic stem cell research, and I am.

RIGHT TO RECOVER—*Yvonne Perry*

- I keep hearing that new discoveries might end the controversy over stem cell research. I wonder if this is true.

- I think that anyone who is against any type of research that would help find cures or treatments for any illness is a selfish, cold-hearted, mean-spirited person who is not a member of the human race.

- I think that we need to educate people on what EXACTLY stem cell research is. People are making the same uninformed, closed-minded decision that could be related to when the birth control pill came out. Then, it was considered abortion. Now, we are educated.

- I think the public needs to be more educated. I also think it needs to be explained of what advantages you get with embryo stem research versus using the umbilical cord. I know in my mind that there are many advantages to stem cell research but it has never been clearly explained if it makes a difference where the stem cells come from.

- I wish more people were more concerned about the quality of life of a human being who is already born - instead of being preoccupied with the "life" of an embryo.

- I would like to have more information on this subject. I'm for any research that will save a life. However, if the government has any control over it then it becomes costly and no accountability.

- I'm a ventilator-dependent quadriplegic. If the stem cells are taken from an umbilical cord or amniotic fluid and not a fetus I am pro stem cell research, if not I'm against it. I'll happily remain in my condition. So my answers were not just yes or no. It depends on where the cells come from.

- It is my opinion that in God's eyes, stem cell research is wrong. We must obey God.

- It is unconscionable to hold up the science that could provide cures for so many people suffering debilitating and deadly medical conditions. Medical waste ought to be recycled to become life's treasure.

- It needs to presented truthfully without political and religious beliefs.

- Killing potential human beings is never an option, especially when so much more promise and remarkable results have been had with adult stem cells. Anyone with a contrary view is in grave denial and their immortal soul is in danger.

- Our government funds many, many inane research projects that make little (if any) contribution to moving the human race forward. It's amazing to me that we would get so self-righteous about stem cell research. My ophthalmologist has been making remarkable strides in treating traumatic blindness with embryonic tissue (donated by mothers after delivery). Why can't we do other projects with that kind of research and completely bypass the 'moral/ethical' considerations? No embryos are used in gathering this tissue. Even if we can't find other ways to utilize post-partum embryonic tissue, I still support stem cell research. Do we have a choice supporting a war that has already killed thousands and has no resolution; approving a government contract that pays $700 for toilet seats; or funding stem cell research? I'll take the research. It strikes me as a more intelligent and humane way to build the future.

- Our motives matter more than our actions because God looks on our heart. Knowing that embryonic stem cell research has the potential to save lives, our intentions in this matter are honorable. Preserving life and promoting human health are among the most precious of values in both Jewish and Christian traditions.

- Please distinguish adult stem cell research is CURING, embryonic is causing tumors.

- Politicians are generally ignorant of science and therefore continue to screw around with other peoples lives.

- Recent medical history reveals that most of the breakthroughs come from privately/corporately funded research labs. From what I understand, it's not an issue of whether the government should fund this research as much as it is an issue of legislation that such research should be allowed.

- See that it is still an embryo thus this is my problem with it. Until it can be proven that this is not a human life I have to be against it. Hopefully the amniotic fluid stem cells will show promise or maybe cord blood stem cells will go on to treat more disorders.

- So much has been done with umbilical cord blood, amniotic fluid, and adult stem cells, why risk the life of an embryo?

- Some of the questions I clicked no on because I did not agree with either answer. This may skew your results.

- Stem Cell is sent and created by GOD for his glory and should be embraced and studied to get people well of literally hundreds of debilitating diseases. People are so mislead by our government and media. THEY JUST DON'T KNOW THE FACTS and it is such a shame.

- Stem cells can be collected from embryonic fluid when babies are born...Stem cell research shows a great deal of potential for treatment of some of life's very worse diseased or injury.

- The government funds numerous frivolous projects. This issue should be clearly researched and funding given if the preliminary tests show promise for improving the health status of ill patients.

- There are many ways to utilize already available cells. Abortions may be one route. At least the option should be available to the woman if she wants to donate. Too much control of OUR bodies. There are possibilities out there if only the religion were taken out of it. Live and let live and perhaps many more can in a better fashion.

- This is important for people for so many reasons. Let's help people that are already alive and not worry so much about cells in a Petri dish.

- To NOT fund and encourage stem cell research of any kind is ignorant and regressive. My hope is that soon we will reach an enlightened state that enables us to truly care for each other and for future generations.

- Too much good could be done for spinal cord injuries, diseases, organ replacements, etc. to not fund this research.

- Try being a cancer patient or paralyzed patient with little hope of survival...we have got to research any possibility for treatments and cures that can help!!!

- We all know who is really behind NOT wanting stem cell research done. It is time. There could be many lives that can be saved!

- We've lost so much time because of the Bush administration and the outright lies concerning this research from the religious right.

- While I am a Christian, I do NOT believe that an embryo is a living being. Therefore I feel the government should provide funding for research done on blastocyst stem cells.

These are some very eye-opening comments about the way Americans view blastocyst stem cell research! Notice that more than half the responders to my survey base their opinion about blastocyst stem cell research on what they've heard in the media. Sixty-seven percent of the responders to my survey claim to be Christians and yet the results show 77.6 percent of them disagree with the president's belief that an embryo is destroyed through blastocyst research. Ninety-two percent of those who took my survey believe blastocystic stem cell research may provide cures for disease or injury but only 76 percent are willing to help fund it.

If you would like to give your personal opinion about blastocyst stem cell research, go to www.right2recover.com and participate in the survey I have set up online. Your comments will remain anonymous and I reserve the right to include the answers in any future book I write or any update I post on my Web site.

Chapter Ten

THE SIGNIFICANCE OF FEDERAL FUNDING

The debate over stem cell research is not really about embryos being destroyed. I have shown sufficient proof that the cells of a blastocyst created in a lab are not a human being; these cells have the potential to be any type of cell under natural or manipulated conditions.

The debate is not whether research using blastocysts should be allowed. The debate is whether blastocyst stem cell research should be financed with the federal taxpayers' dollars.

How Important is Federal Funding for IV-B Research?

The private sector has been funding the research under restrictive conditions for years, and, while we have seen tremendous progress, a lack of greater funds definitely limits advancement toward a cure. Scientists are still in the trial and error stages of working with blastocyst stem cells. Compare that to the medical technology we now have available with adult and cord blood stem cells and you will see how much government funding helps in developing new treatments for disease.

Federal funding will allow more scientists around the world, including our nation's most prominent researchers, to conduct research that will hasten the discovery of therapies, drugs, and treatments for a gamut of illnesses and injuries. Federal funding will ensure collaboration and information sharing among researchers and will lessen the overall costs of doing research. Efforts would no longer need to be duplicated in separate labs that isolate research conducted through federal funds from research conducted through private funding.

H.R. 810

While the stem cell research bill (H.R. 810) that President Bush vetoed in 2006 was not a "be all, do all, end all" solution to the funding situation, it had great potential to at least get the ball rolling. Before we go any farther, let's look at the actual language of H.R. 810, also known as the Stem Cell Research Enhancement Act of 2005.[48]

One Hundred Ninth Congress of the United States of America AT THE SECOND SESSION held at the City of Washington on Tuesday, the third day of January, two thousand and six An Act To amend the Public Health Service Act to provide for human embryonic stem cell research.

Be it enacted by the Senate and House of Representatives of the United States of America in Congress assembled,

SECTION 1. SHORT TITLE.

This Act may be cited as the "Stem Cell Research Enhancement Act of 2005".

SEC. 2. HUMAN EMBRYONIC STEM CELL

RESEARCH.

Part H of title IV of the Public Health Service Act (42 USC. 289 et seq.) is amended by inserting after section 498C the following:

SEC. 498D. HUMAN EMBRYONIC STEM CELL RESEARCH.

(a) In General- Notwithstanding any other provision of law (including any regulation or guidance), the Secretary shall conduct and support research that utilizes human embryonic stem cells in accordance with this section (regardless of the date on which the stem cells were derived from a human embryo).

(b) Ethical Requirements- Human embryonic stem cells shall be eligible for use in any research conducted or supported by the Secretary if the cells meet each of the following:

(1) The stem cells were derived from human embryos that have been donated from in vitro fertilization clinics, were created for the purposes of fertility treatment, and were in excess of the clinical need of the individuals seeking such treatment.

(2) Prior to the consideration of embryo donation and through consultation with the individuals seeking fertility treatment, it was determined that the embryos would never be implanted in a woman and would otherwise be discarded.

(3) The individuals seeking fertility treatment donated the embryos with written informed consent and without receiving any financial or other inducements to make the donation.

(c) Guidelines- Not later than 60 days after the date of the enactment of this section, the Secretary, in consultation with

200

RIGHT TO RECOVER—*Yvonne Perry*

the Director of NIH, shall issue final guidelines to carry out this section.

(d) Reporting Requirements- The Secretary shall annually prepare and submit to the appropriate committees of the Congress a report describing the activities carried out under this section during the preceding fiscal year, and including a description of whether and to what extent research under subsection (a) has been conducted in accordance with this section.

H.R. 810 would have released hundreds of new lines of IV-B stem cells to be used for research regardless of the date they were fertilized. Why is this important? Scientists don't need a higher quantity of cells; they need higher quality cells. As you know, many of the "Bush-approved" lines have been contaminated with mouse feeder cells and cannot be used for research on humans. The technology used for harvesting blastocyst stem cells has improved greatly since 2001.

H.R. 810 would have given researchers access to higher quality cultures than those fertilized prior to August 9, 2001. The newer cell lines would not have animal feeders. Researchers say that the Bush-approved lines are hard to work with, and most stem cell researchers won't bother trying to grow new lines from them in the lab. The knowledge of how to work with the old lines is obsolete, and researchers who are new to this field do not have the "old" knowledge. Instead, they possess cutting-edge and up-to-date skills in working with newer lines that are easier to work with because they renew more quickly for reproducibility. These new lines would include diversity in race and genetic types.

What is so significant about a date? If the U.S. is willing to fund research on a limited number- of IV-Bs, then why not fund research on all of them?

RIGHT TO RECOVER—*Yvonne Perry*

While the federal government does not explicitly prohibit blastocyst stem cell research, it does not officially encourage it, either. Any government decision to fund an activity officially declares national endorsement of the cause. The fact that many state governments have passed legislature that will use state funds for IV-B stem cell research shows that the general public does endorse it. We simply have to convince at least 67 members of Congress to vote according to the wishes of the majority of U.S. citizens. With a two-thirds vote, the President cannot veto the bill. In April 2007, S. 5, the Stem Cell Research Enhancement Act only had 63 in favor—four short of veto-proof status.

The U.S. has long held scientific research in high regard. We already have many programs in place, costing hundreds of billions of dollars, designed to improve the social conditions and medical health of the American people. We all know someone who benefits from Medicaid and Medicare; and undoubtedly we know someone who might benefit from a treatment found through blastocystic stem cell research. All taxpayers would also benefit from federal funding for science that would increase human knowledge, health, and happiness.

Living under majority rule means there are times when we will be the minority and must endure the wishes of the majority even if we don't agree with them. In a letter to President Bush, Iranian President, Mahmoud Ahmadinejad, showed a thread of common sense when he asked:

> *Would it not be more beneficial to bring the U.S. officers and soldiers home, and (than) to spend the astronomical U.S. military expenditures in Iraq for the welfare and prosperity of the American people? As you know very well, many victims of Katrina continue*

to suffer, and countless Americans continue to live in poverty and homelessness.[49]

I am deeply opposed to the war in Iraq, yet my tax dollars are helping pay for the killing of innocent people. I pay federal taxes to support programs that do not benefit me, and I have no choice in the matter. I have to pay Social Security taxes knowing that I may never see a dime of this money when I retire. Why? Because the law requires that I pay for government programs that are for the good of the majority of citizens. Blastocystic stem cell research is for the good of the majority of citizens. Therefore, the government should pay for all types of stem cell technology to be developed, not just some of them.

When Bush vetoed H.R. 810 to expand federal funding for IV-B research, he supported his reason by saying U.S. taxpayers who object to such research should not have to pay for it. In that case, please take me off the Social Security roster! I object and would rather invest my money in other ways.

The only way we are going to discover the potential contained in blastocyst stem cell technology is to allow research to take place, and that requires many funds that could be appropriated from government programs that are wasting taxpayers' money.

Current Federal Law and Policy on Stem Cell Research

On August 9, 2001, Bush announced his policy regarding stem cell research:

> *As a result of private research, more than 60 genetically diverse stem cell lines already exist. I have concluded that we should allow federal funds to be used for research on these existing stem cell lines where the life and death decision has already been made. This*

allows us to explore the promise and potential of stem cell research without crossing a fundamental moral line by providing taxpayer funding that would sanction or encourage further destruction of human embryos that have at least the potential for life.[50]

Prior to 2001, all research on IV-B was conducted through the private sector or in university laboratories using private funds. Even though President Bush's policy regarding blastocyst stem cell research is very restrictive, it does release some federal funds for blastocyst research on stem cell lines created prior to 2001. Thankfully, the current policy allows work supported by private funds to proceed without restriction. These are not the only terms by which federal funding policy are conceived or measured. The policy on the funding of blastocyst stem cell research also rests upon The Dickey Amendment, which the President is required to enforce.

The National Institutes of Health, (NIH) administers most of the federal funding of biomedical research, and is expected to make effective use of those funds through policies that are in place. The NIH devoted over $170 million to the study of human adult stem cells in fiscal year 2002, and approximately $181.5 million in fiscal year 2003. This is about ten times the amount devoted to human blastocystic stem cell research. Other than honoring the usual human subject protections and clinical research requirements, there are no restrictions on what research American scientists can do with adult stem cells using taxpayer funds because these cells are considered to be like any other cells in the body. However, when it comes to a blastocyst stem cell, there are a number of limitations in place. So, what are the policies currently in place regarding IV-B research?

RIGHT TO RECOVER—*Yvonne Perry*

The policy President Bush refers to states that federal funds will only be used for research on existing stem cell lines that were derived with the informed consent of the donors; from excess embryos created solely for reproductive purposes prior to August 9, 2001; and without any financial inducements to the donors. No stem cell lines may be created for research purposes only; they have to be leftover from *in vitro* production for couples who no longer need them for reproductive purposes. Additionally, federal funds would not be used for cloning human blastocyst stem cells for any purpose. Does this mean therapeutic or reproductive cloning, or both types? Does President Bush even know the difference?

President Bush created a President's Council on Bioethics consisting of 18 people to study and advise him regarding embryonic stem cell research, assisted reproduction, cloning, genetic screening, gene therapy, euthanasia, psychoactive drugs, and brain implants among other things. President Clinton had his own Bioethics Council. The key to what decisions are rendered is determined by who sits on this council. Elizabeth Blackburn, the only stem cell biologist on the President's Council on Bioethics, was "fired" from her position when she told her fellow council members that developments in the field of blastocystic stem cells held great promise in the healthcare field. Blackburn and another scientist were replaced with three people having more conservative views.

Determining the eligibility of an IV-B stem cell line for distribution to researchers involves a lengthy process of growth, characterization, quality control and assurance, development, and distribution. Once a line is considered eligible, the negotiation process begins with the companies or institutions owning the cell lines. To ensure that no market develops for human tissue or blastocysts, women or couples who donate eggs or sperm are not to be paid for their contribution. This also keeps individuals from being financially motivated to donate material. This same human material can be sold by fertility labs to research companies. Additional things such as ownership of the treatments or techniques discovered as a result of research, and guidelines for proper use of the cell lines have to be negotiated. This could take more than a year for one cell line. As of September 2003, the owners of the available lines have distributed over 300 shipments of lines to researchers.

In an effort to make more of the eligible lines available, the NIH has created awards as an incentive for stem cell providers to expand, test, and perform quality assurance, and improve distribution of cell lines that meet the NIH's funding criteria. One problem facing the research funding process is a lack of trained researchers who have the skills and techniques to culture human blastocyst stem cells. The lack of personnel is directly connected to the scarcity of funds for IV-B stem cell research. Also, the political and religious controversy surrounding the issue causes some potential researchers to stay away from the field.

Current NIH Director, Dr. Elias A. Zerhouni, said, "I don't think the limiting factor is the cell lines. I really don't. I really think the limiting factor is human capital and trained human capital that can quickly evaluate a wide range of research avenues in stem cells. Therefore, some of the federal funding will need to go for training of new researchers in stem cell culture techniques and to create monetary incentives to lure researchers into a career in this field."

Why Not Use Only Private Funds for IV-B Stem Cell Research?

The current restrictions on federal funds and the controversy surrounding IV-B stem cell research discourage some potential investors from donating funds for blastocystic stem cell research. However, data from 2002 shows that approximately 30 companies in the United States employing more than 1,000 scientists were actively engaged in IV-B stem cell research. Cumulative spending was estimated at $208 million with Geron Corporation alone spending more than $70 million on IV-B stem cell research in 2003. But, where is the oversight committee? Who is making sure the research is adhering to guidelines? Government-funded research has those two important items in place through the NIH.

James Batty, former chairman of the stem cell task force at the U.S. National Institutes of Health, believes publicly funded U.S. researchers have what they need to conduct research on IV-B stem cells. Current Bush-appointed head of the NIH, Dr. Elias Zerhouni, disagrees.

At a hearing about the NIH, an astonishing conversation took place between Senator Tom Harkin (a long-time supporter of IV-B stem cell research) and Dr. Zerhouni.[51] Senator Harkin asked Dr. Zerhouni if scientists would have a better chance of finding new cures or interventions for diseases if the current restrictions on IV-B stem cell research were lifted. Dr. Zerhouni affirmed that the Bush-approved cell lines are not sufficient to do all the research needing to be done. He believes American science and the nation would be better served if scientists had access to cell lines that have emerged since 2001.

Dr. Zerhouni also thinks the claim that adult stem cells are able to do all that blastocyst stem cells can do is overstated.

"The presentations about adult stem cells having as much or more potential than embryonic stem cells, in my view, do not hold scientific water...I think scientists who work in adult stem cells themselves will tell you that we need to pursue as vigorously embryonic stem cells."

Dr. Zerhouni agrees that all angles in stem cell research should be pursued. The fundamental challenge in stem cell research is not just to replace things, like in adult stem cell transplantation. He feels that blastocyst stem cells will help us understand for the first time in the history of mankind how DNA is programmed to reprogram. But, to do that, we need programmed cells (adult) as well as undifferentiated blastocyst cells. "So from my standpoint as NIH director," Dr. Zerhouni says, "it is in the best interest of our scientists, our science and our country that we find ways and the nation finds a way to allow the science to go full speed across adult and embryonic stem cells equally."

Ideally, blastocyst stem cell research should have the opportunity to benefit from both federal and private funds, but doing so has its own complications. The University of Minnesota receives both private and federal funding for IV-B stem cell research. Researchers use Paper Mate Flexgrips in the lab that is federally funded, while researchers in the identical lab across the hall use Uni-ball pens for research that is privately funded. And it's not just about pens. The two laboratories each have their own test tubes, freezers, and microscopes and each maintains elaborate systems to keep their work completely separate. The University of California, San Francisco, reconstructed a laboratory originally financed with U.S. government grants so they could utilize it for stem cell research using $6 million in privately donated money. They also have a lab in the same building where they conduct nearly identical experiments.

However, graduate students are banned from collaborating with one another about what goes on in the other lab.

Dr. John D. Gearhart's research is funded not only by Johns Hopkins, but also privately by Geron Corp. and a patient's group called Project ALS. Gearhart's biggest frustration over the separation of public and private funding is not being able to share discoveries and research information with other researchers. Gearhart says, "It's difficult going to meetings because of the proprietary issues of how much to tell my colleagues."

Having to be concerned with issues of ownership, patents, intellectual property, and proprietary information only serves to slow things down and make the research more costly. The same research has to be done twice—once in a lab supplied with federal dollars and again in a lab supplied by private funds simply because researchers are not allowed to work together on projects. They can compare notes in what is known as the "bright line" in the lab, but all time sheets and expenditures must correspond to the percentage of work done with NIH funds versus non-NIH funds.

Issues with proprietary or intellectual property (IP) rights are also separated according to who funds them. Privately-owned companies hold patent rights to research they have funded with private money. For example, the Wisconsin Alumni Research Foundation (WARF) requires royalty payments from any proceeds from "commercially used" technology derived from IV-B stem cell research done in their lab. They have also exclusively sub-licensed rights to commercialization for therapies for diabetes, heart disease, and central nervous system conditions to Geron Corp. Currently, the NIH is a major player in the IP battle against the constraining patent positions held by WARF. WARF is not alone; Advanced Cell Technology holds a similarly strong patent position on SCNT.

A violation of federal policy would cause the university to be legally responsible for criminal and civil penalties, and even one mistake could endanger federal grants for the lab and the university. Dr. John Boockvar, who heads Cornell University's Neurosurgery Laboratory for Translational Stem Cell Research believes the compliance red tape is a pain in the neck because it only makes the research more difficult. Why are U.S. researchers put at such a disadvantage?

It is my hope that this book will help people understand the facts and fallacies about IV-B stem cell research, and that they will urge their senators to vote for any legislation to allow federal funding for all types of stem cell research.

The Use of Cord Blood

Once considered medical garbage, cord blood was typically thrown away after the mother gave birth. Today, thanks to blood banks and public awareness about treatments using the blood-forming stem cells in cord blood, more and more parents are saving their baby's umbilical cord blood at birth.

According to research in the Journal of Pediatric Hematology/ Oncology, the odds that a child will need to use his or her own stem cells by age twenty-one for current treatments are about 1:2,700, and the odds that a family member would need to use those cells are about 1:1,400. Those are not very high odds, but parents never know when their newborn may need a dose of his own stem cells within the first few years of life.

Private and Public Cord Blood Banking

Both private and public cord banks can store cord blood. A private bank will assure that no one else has access to or utilizes your baby's cord blood without your permission. Costs range from $1,000 to $2,000 for collection and approximately $125 per year for storage. Neither fee is covered by insurance.

Public cord blood banks do not charge the donor for collecting or storing a donation. Public cord blood banks are used to further the research of the medical treatments derived from umbilical cord blood stem cells. These banks supply hospitals with stem cells to use for transplants of non-relatives. Therefore, if you need to access your child's cord blood in the future, there's no assurance that your child's particular blood could be located. Since there is usually enough cord blood collected, it is wise to utilize both private and public blood banks for your baby's cord blood.

Stem Cell Research on Amniotic Fluid

On January 8, 2007, researchers at Wake Forest University and Harvard University reported that they had found a plentiful source of stem cells in the amniotic fluid that cushions babies in the womb. They have produced several different tissue cell types including brain, liver, and bone from cells they drew from amniotic fluid of pregnant women.

While amniotic stem cells can generate a broad range of important cell types, they may not be able to do everything IV-B stem cells can. Scientists do not know exactly how many different cell types can be made from the stem cells found in amniotic fluid. Dr. Anthony Atala, leading researcher for the amniotic fluid study at Wake Forest University in Winston-Salem, North Carolina, hopes these cells will provide a valuable resource for tissue repair and for engineered organs to be medically useful as replacement parts. Atala and his team have already manufactured seven bladders using live tissue grown in the lab. Preliminary tests on humans are still years away. However, Atala does not believe amniotic stem cells should replace blastocyst stem cell research. "Some may be interpreting my research as a substitute for...embryonic stem cells," said Dr. Atala. "I disagree with that... It is essential that National Institutes of Health-funded researchers are able to fully pursue embryonic stem cell research..."[52]

Harvard University stem cell researcher Dr. George Daley believes there is a possibility that the day will come when "expectant parents can freeze amniotic stem cells for future tissue replacement in a sick child without fear of immune rejection." Daley also said:

The discovery shouldn't be used as a replacement for human embryonic stem cell research. While they are fascinating subjects of study in their own right, they are not a substitute for human embryonic stem cells, which allow scientists to address a host of other interesting questions in early human development.[53]

Why Not Use Only Cord Blood, Amniotic Fluid, and Bone Marrow?

If cord blood, amniotic fluid, and bone marrow contain stem cells, why do we need research on blastocyst stem cells? The simple truth is there are no substitutes. While cord blood, amniotic fluid, adult stem cells, reprogramming of cells and other alternate research certainly deserve study, no credible expert supports using them as a replacement for IV-B stem cells.

There are no moral issues attached to the use of cord blood and amniotic fluid, but like adult stem cells, these have already differentiated and have different characteristics than IV-B stem cells. Days-old blastocyst stem cells allow a range of research on the very earliest stages of human development and are more versatile than adult stem cells or fetal cells extracted months later from amniotic fluid or from cord blood at birth.

Sticking a needle into a pregnant woman's uterus can be dangerous. One in 100 amniocentesis results in harm to the developing fetus or mother. Therefore, this is not a safe method for obtaining stem cells, regardless of what kind of organs can be grown from them. Amniotic stem cells are not a replacement for blastocyst stem cells.

Comparing IV-B Stem Cells with Adult Stem Cells

Scientists are still trying to discover which set of stem cell characteristics will ultimately be needed to cure or treat certain diseases. Here are a few key features we know about IV-B stem cells and multipotent progenitor or adult stem cells (ASC):

- IV-B stem cells are indefinite, robust, and self-renewable. IV-B stem cells can transform into virtually any type of cell of the body. Pluripotency disappears as differentiation occurs and development continues.

- ASCs are limited in the number of cells they are able to transform into; in other words, they can only create more of the same type of cells as they already are. For that reason, adult cells are not able to do the same things as IV-B stem cells, which have the characteristics researchers believe are needed to cure some diseases.

- Stem cells exist in relatively large numbers in IV-Bs.

- ASC or multipotent progenitor stem cells have not yet been found in all tissues of the body. In fact, they are scarce in the brain. If neural stem cells are needed, they must be generated from blastocyst stem cells. Bone marrow stem cells must be revved up with medication to stimulate their growth before they can be used for transplantation in the treatment of cancer.

Any knowledge gained from blastocyst stem cells will complement studies of adult and all other types of stem cells, and vice versa. Most scientists agree that therapy advances will be found by responsibly investigating all aspects of stem cell biology.

Federal funding for all types of stem cell research will hasten the scientific progress needed in finding cures for a multitude of illnesses and injuries. Private funding confined to the for-profit, commercial sector means research is being conducted without federal oversight but in accordance with federal laws. If the government funds blastocyst stem cell research, it will also provide oversight of the work and ensure that the research complies with ethical guidelines.

Blastocyst stem cell research should be pursued in three ways:

- Ethically (by abiding by the *Guidelines for Human Embryonic Stem Cell Research* or another mutually agreed upon set of standards that insure proper donor consent, legitimate use of stem cells, and proper creation and storage of stem cell lines)

- Cost-effectively (with accountability for how funds are spent)

- Efficiently (with researchers working together and sharing data to facilitate the advancement of knowledge and discoveries)

There's no doubt that the majority of U.S. citizens who want federal funding for blastocyst stem cell research will win in the end, no matter how strong a battle wages against this technology. It is time to ditch the stem cell debate and begin focusing on what the majority of Americans want regarding how this research should be financed and conducted. It's time to de-politicize stem cell biology.

I'll end this chapter with a quote from Dr. John Kessler:

Like all crusaders, the vocal minority against stem-cell research seeks to impose its beliefs on everyone and to impede (and even imprison) stem-cell researchers. Ironically, in my heart I believe that when stem-cell therapies become a reality, many of the opponents of stem-cell research would eagerly seek any such therapies that could help a beloved family member or friend who was touched by disease. By allowing and supporting stem-cell research in the United States, we will facilitate its progress, keep our researchers within the country and bring stem-cell therapies closer to reality.[54]

Chapter Eleven

CHALLENGING
THE PRENTICE LIST

What is the "Prentice List"? It is a list of fifty-eight to one hundred alleged cures, treatments, or "improvements" misleadlingly attributed to adult stem cells research. The source of this list is an employee of a religious right lobbying group.

First of all, there is a huge difference between people of faith and those known as the "religious right." Religious right groups have an agenda to moralize society by force, using government edicts to impose their ideology on everyone. Not only have they been able to sell their provacative misrepresentation that blastocyst stem cell research kills babies, which it clearly does not, but they are also attempting to "prove" that blastocyst stem cell research has no potential to provide treatments for diseases and injuries, which they very well may. They want us to believe that cord blood, amniotic fluid, and bone marrow have benefits equal to those derived from IV-Bs.

Blastocyst stem cell research is a new field that has not yet entered the human clinical trial stage. No research can be said to be beneficial or harmful until it has been tested and either approved or disapproved for general use. Until human trials are conducted, the assumption that IV-B stem cells have not presented any useful treatment is not valid.

Groups in Opposition

The debate over the merits and morality of blastocyst stem cell research is fueled by a small but verbal minority attempting to delay funding. A list found in a Legislative Bulletin in May of 2005 provided by a Republican study committee chaired by Representative Jeb Hensnarling of Texas named 17 groups in opposition to H.R. 810 (Stem Cell Research Enhancement Act of 2005). These same groups are opposed to H.R. 3 (Stem Cell Research Enhancement Act of 2007).

It's interesting to note that not one medical research institution, medical school, patient advocacy group, disease foundation, or disease-specific charity opposes the research.[55]

What groups do make up the opposition? Thirteen of the seventeen groups are conservative religious lobbying organizations:

1. Center for Reclaiming America (started by evangelist D. James Kennedy)
2. Christian Coalition
3. Christian Medical Association
4. Concerned Women for America
5. Coral Ridge Ministries (D. James Kennedy)
6. Cornerstone Policy Research (possibly defunct)
7. Culture of Life Foundation
8. Family Research Council (started by James Dobson, this group employs David Prentice). The FRC is a tax exempt organization - Section 170 of Internal Revenue Code

9. Focus on the Family (James Dobson)
10. Religious Freedom Coalition
11. Southern Baptist Convention
12. Traditional Values Coalition
13. U.S. Conference of Catholic Bishops

Four of the 17 groups are anti-abortionist groups: Eagle Forum (started by conservative activist Phyllis Schlafly, who led opposition to the Equal Rights Amendment); National Right to Life Committee; Republican National Committee for Life; and Susan B. Anthony List.

A similar and perhaps related group, the Family Bioethics Counsel,engaged in legal proceedings to shut down California's new stem cell program. Groups like these, while they may be well-intentioned and truly believe they are saving embryos, are doing far more harm than good.

Senator Brownback and the Family Research Council

U.S. Senator Sam Brownback (R-KS) and other opponents of blastocyst stem cell research claim there are between 65 and 72 human illnesses (including Parkinson's, Sandhoff disease and spinal cord injury) that can be successfully cured or treated with adult stem cells. Claims such as these are misleading and disappointing at best. Do you know of anyone with spinal cord injury who has been treated with adult stem cells and recovered completely? If I did, I wouldn't have written this book. The cure would be available and people would be waiting in line to be treated.

The list of such illnesses was created by blastocyst stem cell research opponent David A. Prentice of the religious right's Family Research Council, the powerful lobbying group that advises Senator

Brownback. The number of alleged "cures" varies in number from 58-100 depending on the speaker, which could be anyone from an anti-science Congressional representative seeking justification for blocking life-saving research, to supposed "science" writers like Michael Fumento. Prentice himself claims 72 "improvements in the real lives of patients," but the list is frequently offered as outright cures.

Legitimate adult stem cell research has been ongoing for approximately half a century. Despite a multi-decade head start over blastocyst stem cell research, adult stem cells have been shown to improve only about nine conditions on the Prentice list. Only nine conditions on the Prentice list have demonstrated both safety and efficacy in all three phases of clinical trials and are considered as "standard therapy" by the U.S. Food and Drug Administration (FDA) treatments. These nine are:

1. Acute Lymphoblastic Leukemia
2. Acute Myelogenous Leukemia
3. Aplastic Anemia
4. Chronic Myelogenous Leukemia
5. Juvenile Myelomonocytic Leukemia
6. Multiple Myeloma
7. Myelodysplasia
8. Severe Combined Immunodeficiency Syndrome-X1
9. Thalassemia Major

Fortunately, the truth about adult stem cells (ASC) has been revealed. While a valuable tool in its own right, ASC are in no way a substitute for the greater potential of blastocystic therapies.

The Prentice List Examined

Shane G. Smith, Ph.D. is the Science Director of the Children's Neurobiological Solutions Foundation (CNS Foundation). In 2004, Shane served as Science Director for California's successful *Yes on Proposition 71,* the California Stem Cell Research & Cures Initiative campaign. He is also one of the three men who wrote an article that destroys the credibility of the Prentice list.

William Neaves Ph.D. (president of the Stowers Institute for Medical Research), and Steven Teitelbaum M.D. (Wilma and Roswell Messing Professor of Pathology and Immunology at Washington University), and Shane Smith Ph.D published their findings regarding the Prentice list in *Science* in July 2006:

> *The references Prentice cites as the basis for his list include various case reports, a meeting abstract, a newspaper article, and anecdotal testimony before a Congressional committee. A review of those references reveals that Prentice not only misrepresents existing adult stem cell treatments, but also frequently distorts the nature and content of the references he cites. By promoting the falsehood that adult stem cell treatments are already in general use for 65 diseases and injuries, Prentice and those who repeat his claims mislead laypeople and cruelly deceive patients.[56]*

Fabricated Success Stories

"Adult Stem Cells: Nine Faces of Success"—a pamphlet produced and distributed by the Family Research Council—cites several cases of patients said to have been cured by adult stem cells. Interviews with some of the people cited as cured, however, reveal a different story.

In the case of Parkinson's disease (PD), for example, a

single individual, Dennis Turner, is cited as cured. Is he? Let's ask someone who suffers from the cruel disease.

Rayilyn (Ray) Brown is a woman suffering from Parkinson's disease (PD) since 1996. She uses the computer to lobby for blastocyst stem cell research. She and Diane Wyshak, whose son-in-law has diabetes, post regularly on PIEN (Parkinson's Information Exchange Network) to keep people on the list informed. She and Diane offer assistance to letter writing campaigns through online stem cell advocacy sites like SCAN (Stem Cell Action Network) and CAMR (Coalition for Advancement of Medical Research). Ray has talked to the one person supposedly cured of PD by adult stem cells. Sometime in 1999, Dennis Turner had a Deep Brain Stimulation (DBS) surgery wherein Vice President of NeuroGeneration Dr. Michael Levesque of Cedars Sinai in Los Angeles took Turner's neural stem cells, cultivated and expanded them for nine months in a lab and then replanted them in his brain.

It is important to immediately recognize that DBS surgery itself is often used to alleviate some of the symptoms of Parkinson's disease. Here's how it works:

Approved in 1999, DBS surgery is performed while the patient is awake. The head is shaved and put into an iron "halo" to hold it still during the process. A shot of Novocain, a local aesthetic, is given in the scalp before the incision. Two holes are drilled in the skull and a bundle of electrodes is placed in the subthalmic nucleus (STN)—an area of the brain that is over-stimulated in patients with Parkinson's disease. An MRI scan is used to help the surgeon navigate the electrodes. Leads from the electrodes are inserted under the scalp, down the neck, and into the chest. In a separate surgery a "brain pacemaker" that uses wires and a battery source, is installed in the chest. This electronic device is connected to the leads in the brain. A neurologist programs the transmitters to send a continuous but precise electrical current to the brain. Results range from having little influence to restoring one's life to near-normal for a period of months to several years.

Turner's symptoms of Parkinson's disease disappeared for about four or five years after having both DBS surgery and implants of his own brain cells. Having two variables in any scientific experiment makes it impossible to determine which variable caused the effect. Dr. Levesque claims the electrical current to Dennis Turner was never turned on. So it is not known whether DBS or adult stem cells were responsible for Turner's disappearance of symptoms. It is possible that the results were from the DBS surgery and not adult stem cell therapy or vice versa.

Ray wanted to know more and possibly have the treatment herself, so she contacted Dr. Levesque's office in the spring of 2003. She was not encouraged to enter Dr. Levesque's Phase II. In fact, she was warned that there were no guarantees and was gently steered to have DBS surgery. She had a bilateral DBS (with no adult stem cells at all) in June 2003 and a redo in September 2003 by Dr. Thomas Waltz, at Scripps Clinic in La Jolla, California. Both those surgeries successfully controlled her tremors for a time, but nothing else. In fact, the procedure destroyed her voice making it difficult for her to speak.

By March of 2006, Dennis Turner confirmed to Ray that his Parkinson's had returned with a vengeance. However, the January 2007 Family Research Council's pamphlet, "Adult Stem Cell Treatments Nine Faces of Success," still contains Turner's story about how he had been cured by adult stem cell therapy. The White House also produced a pamphlet in January 2007 listing Dennis

Turner as a success story. That pamphlet also included Patricia Payne, a Catholic blastocyst stem cell research opponent, who testified before the Massachusetts State Legislature in February 2005 that she was going to be a participant in Levesque's Phase II. Phase II stopped in July 2005 because Levesque's labs were not up to FDA standards. Therefore, Payne was never in the study, yet she, along with Turner and ten unnamed people in Kentucky, were still listed as adult stem cell success stories in the latest pamphlet. These people received no stem cells of any kind.

I tried to download the "free" pamphlet on FRC's Web site. After having to fill out a form that collected a lot of personal information, I was asked to make a donation. The email I received confirming my registration had no attachment, no link to download the document, and no instructions on how to obtain the pamphlet. Therefore, I was unsuccessful in getting a copy of the pamphlet; however, I did start receiving FRC's newsletter the next day. Fortunately, Ray had an extra copy of the pamphlet and she shared it with me.

The ten unnamed Kentuckians mentioned above were participants in therapy trials with Amgen—a drug maker who created a synthetic form of Glial Cell Line Derived Neurotrophic Factor (GDNF) using recombinant DNA techniques in 1993. GDNF is a naturally occurring protein found in the brain, believed to nourish and promote the growth, regeneration, and protection of dopamine producing neurons. GDNF was delivered to the patients by an infusion pump. While the patients temporarily experienced significant functional improvements while receiving GDNF, we must note that GDNF is *NOT* a stem cell; it is a drug. Amgen terminated all trials and treatments and aborted the study in 2004 because they felt the drug was potentially dangerous.

In early 2006, Ray saw a video of Turner and Levesque's 2004 testimony led by Senator Sam Brownback before a Senate committee depicting the "successes" of adult stem cell treatments. Turner's head was shaking in a manner consistent with PD—he was obviously not cured. If he is not a true success story, why is his story being used to mislead people?

And remember, Dennis Turner is the only individual cited as "cured" of Parkinson's by adult stem cells—in reality neither he nor anybody else has been cured of this dreaded condition, which is all the more reason to go forward with blastocystic research for a cure.

Spinal cord injury? Has that been cured by adult stem cells? Let's take a look at the paralyzed person most publicly cited as having benefited from adult stem cells.

Susan Fajt was in a car accident on November 17, 2001 that severely injured her spine. After six months in a wheelchair, she decided to take her rehab to the next level and began looking for specialists who could help her. She tried treatments at Texas Research and Recovery (TEAR) and traveled all over the world seeking a cure that would restore her mobility. She was willing to try anything in order to be able to walk again. When she heard that adult stem cells might be able to help her, she went to Dr. Carlos Lima through Detroit Medical Center. Dr. Lima is a neurologist at Hospital Egaz Moniz in Lisbon, Portugal who performed surgery on Susan in which she was told that she was receiving adult stem cell transplants in her spine. She later learned that olfactory ensheathing cells, rather than adult stem cells, were used. Wise Young, director of cell biology and neuroscience at Rutgers University, says he is not sure the treatment Fajt received included any adult stem cells at all. He said she received nasal mucosa transplantations into her spinal cord. There was no follow up by Dr. Lima or any of the American doctors who watched as Lima performed the 12-hour surgery.

Susan regained some sensation in her lower extremities after the $30,000 procedure, but nothing useful in terms of function, no controllable movements, nothing close to miraculous. Not satisfied with her recovery, Susan went to Dr. Albert Bohbot, a researcher in France who utilizes laser treatments to address various neurological pathologies. Laserpuncture therapy combines traditional Chinese acupuncture with laser treatment. Using a sophisticated electronic laser device, Dr. Bohbot administered infrared energy to acupuncture meridians to stimulate dermatome levels that affect spinal cord function. After the treatment, Susan regained some control of her bodily functions, but still not the miracle cure she was hoping for. However, she was fitted for leg braces with which she is able to use a walker to move about slowly and methodically. It is important to recognize that many paralytics can "walk" with enormous effort. If their legs are sufficiently braced, they can lean forward with their upper bodies and slowly drag their legs in step-like motions—but this in no way means they are healed.

It was after her treatment in France that Senator Brownback contacted Susan asking her to go before the Senate with him. Feeling like a guinea pig with nothing to lose, she agreed.

However, Susan is upset that a photo of her was used without her permission by Representative Dave Weldon (R-Florida). Senator Weldon used the poster-size photo of himself standing beside Susan, who was wearing braces as she held to a walker, to offer evidence that blastocystic stem cell research was unnecessary since adult stem cells can help severely injured people such as Susan walk again. "This poster is of a young lady who was paralyzed for years and had an adult stem cell transplant," Weldon said. "She is able to stand up."

Members of the House of Representatives were about to vote on a bill that would approve funding for blastocystic stem-cell research. Ms. Fajt, who favors funding of all types of stem cell research, is troubled that SenatorWeldon gave a false impression.

"If Weldon hadn't used my photo to discredit embryonic stem cell research by saying a cure could be found with adult stem cells," said Susan, "the bill might have passed and the research might have been federally funded."

Susan has spoken with Dr. Keirstead who believes researchers are getting closer to moving into clinical trials using IV-B stem cell therapies on humans. She has also been in touch with researchers who are using these therapies on primates recovering from spinal cord injury.

Ms. Fajt wants to live her life with passion and courage, and she truly believes that IV-B stem cell research can come up with a cure or treatment for SCI. "I absolutely know it's doable," Susan told me. "I favor federal funding for all types of stem cell research. I always have, and always will, even if it doesn't help me. It will help someone."

The Adult Stem Cell Success Stories in the 2006 version of the pamphlet claimed that adult stem cells have been used successfully in the treatment of

1. Autoimmune Disease: Multiple Sclerosis, Diabetes, Crohn's, and Lupus
2. Corneal Reconstruction
3. Parkinson's disease
4. Spinal Cord Injuries

5. Heart Tissue Regeneration
6. Anemias, Cancers, and Other Diseases[57]

After numerous email correspondences with UCI anatomy and neurobiology professor, Dr. Fallon, I was almost certain that no approved and effective therapeutic treatments exist for central nervous system damage. While certain types of cancers are treated with adult stem cells from bone marrow or cord blood, the neurological and autoimmune illnesses and injuries on the pamphlet's list have not shown any response to adult stem cells.

I took the above list of claims to Dr. Madan Jagasia, Assistant Professor of Medicine at Vanderbilt University Medical Center, who confirmed, "To my knowledge there are no human studies yet of using adult stem cells to treat the conditions you have mentioned from a regenerative standpoint."

The Prentice list deceives good people who honestly believe that blastocyst stem cell research is morally reprehensible. The impact of false claims regarding the curative power of adult stem cell treatments is devastating. Not only has it offered political cover to opponents of research who have used these claims to say there is no need for any other research, but it may even cause desperate people to go out of the U.S. seeking clinics and unproven treatments that put them in danger.

Why would "Christian" organizations knowingly deceive the public in such a way? And why would the Bush White House not only condone it, but issue more erroneous information to boot?

A Twisted White House Document

A White House document published in January 2007, "Advancing Stem Cell Science without Destroying Human Life" claims new methods of making stem cells render IV-B stem cells obsolete. Are they right?

This 67-page report cites the work of Drs. Kevin Eggan, Chad Cowan, and Douglas Melton regarding reprogramming of adult stem cells. The White House Office of Domestic Policy team did not give the doctors any opportunity to correct the report's clear misrepresentation of their work, which was used to support the false notion that adult stem cells are able to do the same things as blastocyst stem cells.

At a January 19, 2007, hearing, U.S. Senator Tom Harkin (D-IA) had the following response:

> *...the White House released a 60-page polemic against embryonic stem cell research in which it touted research by Kevin Eggan of Harvard, who testified before my subcommittee last year. Here's what Dr. Eggan wrote in response to that White House report: "We are disappointed that the White House Office of Domestic Policy gave us no opportunity to correct the report's clear misrepresentation of our work ...On the contrary, we assert that human embryonic stem cells hold great promise to find new treatments and cures for diseases, and we support ... the Stem Cell Research Enhancement Act."[58]*

Others agree that blastocyst stem cells offer characteristics that adult and amniotic stem cells do not. Dr. Lawrence S. B. Goldstein is Professor of Cellular and Molecular Medicine at the University of California, San Diego, School of Medicine. In an article co-written by Paul Berg and George Q. Daley, dated July 19, 2005, Professor Goldstein said:

> *We want to be very clear: The most successful demonstrated method for creating the most versatile type of stem cells capable of becoming many types of mature human cells is to derive them from human embryos—at present, excess embryos created at in vitro*

fertilization clinics and freely donated for research by couples who choose not to have them destroyed as medical waste.[59]

Regarding the document "Advancing Stem Cell Science without Destroying Human Life" Goldstein said:

> *Although this paper is interesting, I am not convinced that the amniotic stem cells are pluripotent. More work is needed to verify and validate these findings. For my work on human neurons, the amniotic stem cells don't appear to make neurons as usable as what we routinely make with human embryonic stem cells.*[60]

Groups Supporting the Stem Cell Research Enhancement Act

In their opinion editorial dated January 9, 2007, published by St. Louis Post-Dispatch, Drs. Neaves, Teitelbaum, and Smith report:

> *The overwhelming majority of scientists and medical organizations—including the American Medical Association, Association of American Medical Colleges and the National Academies of Science—believe that both adult and embryonic stem cell research should be pursued. These organizations are joined by more than 100 patient groups such as the Juvenile diabetes Research Foundation, the Christopher Reeve Foundation, Parkinson's Action Network and the CNS Foundation.*
>
> *The reason for this scientific consensus is that adult and embryonic stem cells have their own distinct characteristics and their own distinct potential to provide treatments and cures. Those holding this view include many of the researchers into the uses of adult stem cells whose work has been mischaracterized*

by opponents of research using embryonic stem cells. A number of these researchers have signed statements verifying the misrepresentation of their published work and stating their personal support for both embryonic stem cell research and adult stem cell research.

We hope that members of Congress will dismiss the notion that one kind of stem cell research obviates the need for the other and will understand the essential importance of a broad approach to stem cell research.[61]

There are 518 organized groups in favor of overturning the Bush prohibition on federal funding of new stem cell lines. The list below includes patient advocacy groups, health organizations, research universities, scientific societies, religious groups and other interested institutions and associations, representing millions of patients, scientists, health care providers and advocates. I know the list is long, but I want to include it so you may check to see if any of the groups you are affiliated with support H.R.3 –the Stem Cell Enhancement Act of 2007.[62]

1. AAALAC International
2. AARP
3. Acadia Pharmaceuticals
4. Accelerated Cure Project for Multiple Sclerosis
5. Adams County Economic Development, Inc.
6. AdvaMed
7. Affymetrix, Inc.
8. Albert Einstein School of Medicine
9. Allen Institute for Brain Science
10. Alliance for Aging Research

11. Alliance for Lupus Research
12. Alnylam US, Inc.
13. Alpha-1 Foundation
14. ALS Association
15. Ambulatory Pediatric Association
16. America on the Move Foundation
17. American Academy of Nursing
18. American Academy of Pediatric Dentistry
19. American Academy of Pediatrics
20. American Association for Cancer Research
21. American Association for Dental Research
22. American Association for Geriatric Psychiatry
23. American Association for the Advancement of Science
24. American Association of Anatomists
25. American Association of Clinical Endocrinologists
26. American Association of Colleges of Nursing
27. American Association of Colleges of Osteopathic Medicine
28. American Association of Colleges of Pharmacy
29. American Association of Neurological Surgeons/Congress of Neurological Surgeons
30. American Association of Public Health Dentistry
31. American Autoimmune Related Diseases Association
32. American Brain Coalition
33. American Chemical Society
34. American Chronic Pain Association
35. American College of Cardiology
36. American College of Medical Genetics
37. American College of Neuropsychopharmacology
38. American College of Obstetricians and Gynecologists
39. American College of Surgeons

40. American Dental Association
41. American Dental Education Association
42. American Diabetes Association
43. American Federation for Aging Research
44. American Gastroenterological Association
45. American Geriatrics Society
46. American Institute for Medical and Biological Engineering
47. American Institute for Stuttering
48. American Medical Association
49. American Medical Informatics Association
50. American Pain Foundation
51. American Parkinson's Disease Association (Arizona Chapter)
52. American Pediatric Society
53. American Psychiatric Association
54. American Psychological Association
55. American Physiological Society
56. American Public Health Association
57. American Society for Biochemistry and Molecular Biology
58. American Society for Bone and Mineral Research
59. American Society for Cell Biology
60. American Society of Clinical Oncology
61. American Society for Clinical Pathology
62. American Society for Clinical Pharmacology and Therapeutics
63. American Society for Microbiology
64. American Society for Neural Transplantation and Repair
65. American Society for Pharmacology and Experimental Therapeutics
66. American Society for Reproductive Medicine

67. American Society for Therapeutic Radiology and Oncology
68. American Society of Critical Care Anesthesiologists
69. American Society of Hematology
70. American Society of Human Genetics
71. American Society of Nephrology
72. American Society of Tropical Medicine and Hygiene
73. American Sociological Association
74. American Thoracic Society
75. American Thyroid Association
76. American Transplant Foundation
77. Americans for Medical Progress
78. amFAR, The Foundation for AIDS Research
79. APBD Research Foundation
80. ARC of the United States
81. Arizona State University College of Nursing
82. Arthritis Foundation
83. Arthritis Foundation, Rocky Mountain Chapter
84. Association for Clinical Research Training
85. Association for Prevention Teaching and Research
86. Association for Research in Vision and Ophthalmology
87. Association of Academic Health Centers
88. Association of Academic Physiatrists
89. Association of American Cancer Institutes
90. Association of American Medical Colleges
91. Association of American Physicians
92. Association of American Universities
93. Association of American Veterinary Medical Colleges
94. Association of Anatomy, Cell Biology and Neurobiology Chairpersons
95. Association of Anesthesiology Program Directors
96. Association of Black Cardiologists

97. Association of Chairs of Departments of Physiology
98. Association of Independent Research Institutes
99. Association of Medical School Microbiology and Immunology Chairs
100. Association of Medical School Pediatric Department Chairs
101. Association of Medical School Pharmacology Chairs
102. Association of Minority Health Professions Schools
103. Association of Professors of Human and Medical Genetics
104. Association of Professors of Medicine
105. Association of Public Health Laboratories
106. Association of Reproductive Health Professionals
107. Association of Schools and Colleges of Optometry
108. Assurant Health
109. Asthma and Allergy Foundation of America
110. Athena Diagnostics
111. Aurora Economic Development Council
112. Axion Research Foundation
113. Baylor College of Medicine
114. Baylor College of Medicine Graduate School of Biomedical Sciences
115. Beth Israel Deaconess Medical Center
116. Biophysical Society
117. Biotechnology Industry Organization
118. Blood Center of Wisconsin, Inc.
119. B'nai B'rith International
120. Boston University School of Medicine
121. Brigham and Women's Hospital
122. Bristol-Myers Squibb Company
123. Broadened Horizons

124. Brody School of Medicine at East Carolina University
125. Brown University
126. Buck Institute for Age Research
127. Burns & Allen Research Institute
128. Burrill & Company
129. Burroughs Wellcome Fund
130. C3: Colorectal Cancer Coalition
131. California Biomedical Research Association
132. California Institute for Regenerative Medicine
133. California Institute of Technology
134. Californians for Cures
135. Cancer Care
136. Cancer Research and Prevention Foundation
137. CADASIL Together We Have Hope
138. Canon U.S. Life Sciences, Inc.
139. Cardiovascular Research Foundation
140. Case Western Reserve University School of Dentistry
141. Case Western Reserve University School of Medicine
142. Cedars-Sinai Health System
143. Center for Inquiry
144. Center for Information & Study on Clinical Research Participation
145. Center for Global Health and Medical Diplomacy
146. Center for the Advancement of Health
147. CFIDS Association of America
148. Charles R. Drew University of Medicine and Science
149. Charles River Laboratories
150. Child & Adolescent Bipolar Foundation
151. Children's Hospital Boston
152. Children's Memorial Research Center

153. Children's Neurobiological Solutions Foundation
154. Children's Research Institute (Columbus)
155. Children's Research Institute (Washington)
156. Christopher Reeve Foundation
157. City and County of Denver
158. City of Commerce City, CO
159. City of Hope National Medical Center
160. City of Westminster, CO
161. Clinical Research Forum
162. Cold Spring Harbor Laboratory
163. Coleman Institute for Cognitive Disabilities, University of Colorado System
164. Colfax Marathon Partnership, Inc.
165. Colorado Bioscience Association
166. Colorado Office of Economic Development and International Trade
167. Columbia University
168. Community Health Partnership
169. Conference of Boston Teaching Hospitals
170. Connecticut United for Research Excellence, Inc.
171. Coriell Institute for Medical Research
172. Cornell University
173. Council for the Advancement of Nursing Science (CANS)
174. Critical Path Institute (C-Path)
175. CURE (Citizens United for Research in Epilepsy)
176. Cure Alzheimer's Fund
177. CuresNow
178. Cure Paralysis Now
179. Damon Runyon Cancer Research Foundation
180. Dana-Farber Cancer Institute

181. Dartmouth Medical School
182. DENTSPLY International
183. Digene Corporation
184. Disciples for Choice
185. Disciples Justice Action Network
186. Discovery Partners International
187. Doheny Eye Institute
188. Drexel University College of Medicine
189. Drexel University School of Public Health
190. Duke University Medical Center
191. East Tennessee State University James H. Quillen College of Medicine
192. Eli Lilly and Company
193. Elizabeth Glaser Pediatric AIDS Foundation
194. Emory University Nell Hodgson Woodruff School of Nursing
195. Emory University Rollins School of Public Health
196. Emory University School of Medicine
197. The Episcopal Church
198. Equal Partners in Faith
199. Endocrine Society
200. The FAIR Foundation
201. FasterCures
202. FD Hope Foundation
203. Federation of American Societies for Experimental Biology
204. Federation of State Medical Boards of the United States, Inc.
205. Food Allergy Project, Inc.
206. Ford Finance, Inc.

207. Forsyth Institute
208. Fox Chase Cancer Center
209. Fred Hutchinson Cancer Research Center
210. Friends of Cancer Research
211. Friends of the National Institute for Dental and Craniofacial Research
212. Friends of the National Institute of Nursing Research
213. Friends of the National Library of Medicine
214. Genetic Alliance
215. Genetics Policy Institute
216. George Mason University
217. Gilda's Club Worldwide
218. GlaxoSmithKline
219. Guillain Barre Syndrome Foundation International
220. Gynecologic Cancer Foundation
221. Hadassah
222. Harvard University
223. Hereditary Disease Foundation
224. HHT Foundation International, Inc.
225. Home Safety Council
226. Howard University College of Dentistry
227. Howard University College of Medicine
228. IBM Life Sciences Division
229. Illinois State University Mennonite College of Nursing
230. ImmunoGen, Inc.
231. Indiana University
232. Indiana University School of Medicine
233. Infectious Diseases Society of America
234. Institute for Systems Biology
235. Intercultural Cancer Council Caucus

236. International Foundation for Anticancer Drug Discovery (IFADD)
237. International Longevity Center – USA
238. International Myeloma Foundation
239. International Society for Stem Cell Research
240. Invitrogen Corporation
241. Iraq Veterans for a Cure
242. Iron Disorders Institute
243. The J. David Gladstone Institutes
244. Jefferson Economic Council
245. Jeffrey Modell Foundation
246. Jewish Council for Public Affairs
247. Jewish Women International
248. Johns Hopkins Institutions
249. Johnson & Johnson
250. Joint Commission on Accreditation of Healthcare Organizations (JCAHO)
251. Juvenile diabetes Research Foundation
252. Keck School of Medicine of the University of Southern California
253. Keystone Symposia on Molecular and Cellular Biology
254. KID Foundation
255. Kidney Cancer Association
256. La Jolla Institute for Allergy and Immunology
257. Lance Armstrong Foundation
258. Lawson Wilkins Pediatric Endocrine Society
259. Lehigh Valley Hospital and Health Network
260. Leukemia & Lymphoma Society
261. Los Angeles Biomedical Research Institute at Harbor-UCLA Medical Center

262. Louisiana State University Health Sciences Center
263. Louisiana State University HSC School of Dentistry
264. Lovelace Respiratory Research Institute
265. Lung Cancer Alliance
266. Lupus Foundation of America, Inc.
267. Lupus Research Institute
268. Lymphatic Research Foundation
269. Lymphoma Research Foundation
270. Malecare Prostate Cancer Support
271. Marine Biological Laboratory
272. Masonic Medical Research Laboratory
273. Massachusetts Biotechnology Council
274. Massachusetts General Hospital
275. Massachusetts Institute of Technology
276. MaxCyte, Inc.
277. Mayo Clinic
278. McLaughlin Research Institute
279. Medical College of Georgia
280. The Medical Foundation, Inc.
281. Medical University of South Carolina
282. MedStar Research Institute (MRI)
283. Meharry Medical College School of Dentistry
284. Memorial Sloan-Kettering Cancer Center
285. Memory Pharmaceuticals
286. Mercer University
287. Metro Denver Economic Development Corporation
288. Miami Children's Hospital
289. Morehouse School of Medicine
290. Mount Sinai Medical Center
291. Mount Sinai School of Medicine

292. National Alliance for Eye and Vision Research
293. National Alliance for Hispanic Health
294. National Alliance for Research on Schizophrenia and Depression
295. National Alliance on Mental Illness
296. National Alopecia Areata Foundation
297. National Association for Biomedical Research
298. National Association of State and Land Grant Colleges
299. National Caucus of Basic Biomedical Science Chairs
300. National Coalition for Cancer Survivorship
301. National Coalition for Women with Heart Disease
302. National Council of Jewish Women
303. National Coalition for Cancer Research
304. National Council on Spinal Cord Injury
305. National Down Syndrome Society
306. National Electrical Manufacturers Association
307. National Emphysema/COPD Association
308. National Foundation for Ectodermal Dysplasias
309. National Health Council
310. National Hispanic Health Foundation
311. National Hemophilia Foundation
312. National Jewish Medical and Research Center
313. National Marfan Foundation
314. National Multiple Sclerosis Society
315. National Osteoporosis Foundation
316. National Partnership for Women and Families
317. National Pharmaceutical Council
318. National Prostate Cancer Coalition
319. National Quality Forum
320. National Venture Capital Association

321. Nebraskans for Research
322. Nemours
323. New Jersey Association for Biomedical Research
324. New Jersey Dental School
325. New York Blood Center
326. New York College of Osteopathic Medicine
327. New York Stem Cell Foundation
328. New York University College of Dentistry
329. New York University Medical Center
330. New York-Presbyterian Hospital
331. North American Brain Tumor Coalition
332. North Carolina Association for Biomedical Research
333. Northwest Association for Biomedical Research
334. Northwestern University
335. Nova Southeastern University College of Dental Medicine
336. Novartis Pharmaceuticals
337. Ohio State University
338. Oklahoma Medical Research Foundation
339. Oral Health America
340. Oregon Health & Science University
341. Oregon Health & Science University School of Nursing
342. Oregon Research Institute
343. Oxford Bioscience Partners
344. Pacific Health Research Institute
345. Parent Project Muscular Dystrophy
346. Parkinson's Action Network
347. Parkinson's Disease Foundation
348. Partnership for Prevention
349. Pennsylvania Society for Biomedical Research
350. Pharmaceutical Research and Manufacturers of America

351. Pittsburgh Development Center
352. PRIM&R, Public Responsibility in Medicine & Research
353. Project A.L.S.
354. Prostate Cancer Foundation
355. Quest for the Cure
356. Religious Coalition for Reproductive Choice
357. Rensselaer Polytechnic Institute
358. Research!America
359. Research for Cure
360. Research Foundation for Mental Hygiene, Inc
361. Resolve: The National Infertility Association
362. RetireSafe
363. Rett Syndrome Research Foundation
364. Rice University
365. The Rockefeller University
366. Robert Packard Center for ALS Research at Johns Hopkins
367. Rosalind Franklin University of Medicine and Science
368. Rutgers University
369. Salk Institute for Biological Studies
370. sanofi-aventis
371. Sarcoma Foundation of America
372. The Schepens Eye Research Institute
373. The Scientist
374. Scleroderma Research Foundation
375. The Scripps Research Institute
376. Secular Coalition for America
377. Sjogren's Syndrome Foundation, Inc.
378. S.L.E. Lupus Foundation
379. Sloan-Kettering Institute for Cancer Research
380. The Smith-Kettlewell Eye Research Institute

381. Society for Advancement of Violence and Injury Research (SAVIR)
382. Society for Neuroscience
383. Society for Pediatric Research
384. Society for Women's Health Research
385. Society of Academic Anesthesiology Chairs
386. Society of Gynecologic Oncologists
387. The Society for Investigative Dermatology
388. South Alabama Medical Science Foundation
389. South Dakota State University
390. Southern Illinois University School of Medicine
391. SPARC, The Scholarly Publishing & Academic Resources Coalition
392. Spina Bifida Association of America
393. The Spiral Foundation
394. Stamford Hospital
395. Stanford University
396. State University of New York Downstate Medical Center College of Medicine at Brooklyn
397. State University of New York Upstate Medical University
398. Stem Cell Research Foundation
399. Steven and Michele Kirsch Foundation
400. Stem Cell Action Network
401. Stony Brook University
402. Strategic Health Policy International, Inc.
403. Student Society for Stem Cell Research
404. Suicide Prevention Action Network-USA (SPAN)
405. Take Charge! Cure Parkinson's, Inc.
406. Temple University School of Dentistry
407. Texans for the Advancement of Medical Research

408. Texas A&M University Health Science Center
409. Texas Tech University Health Sciences Center
410. Tourette Syndrome Association
411. Travis Roy Foundation
412. Tufts University
413. Tufts University School of Dental Medicine
414. Tulane University Health Sciences Center
415. Union of Concerned Scientists
416. Unite 2 Fight Paralysis
417. United Church of Christ
418. United Spinal Foundation
419. University at Buffalo; State University of New York
420. University of Alabama at Birmingham School of Medicine
421. University of Alabama at Birmingham School of Nursing
422. University of Alabama at Birmingham School of Public Health
423. University of Arizona College of Medicine
424. University of Arkansas for Medical Sciences
425. University of California, Berkeley
426. University of California, Berkeley School of Public Health
427. University of California, Davis School of Medicine
428. University of California, Irvine School of Medicine
429. University of California, Los Angeles School of Medicine
430. University of California, San Diego School of Medicine/ Health Sciences
431. University of California, San Francisco
432. University of California System
433. University of Chicago
434. University of Cincinnati Medical Center
435. University of Colorado at Denver and Health Sciences Center

436. University of Colorado System
437. University of Connecticut School of Medicine
438. University of Florida
439. University of Florida College of Dentistry
440. University of Georgia
441. University of Illinois
442. University of Iowa
443. University of Kansas
444. University of Kansas Medical Center
445. University of Kansas Medical Center School of Nursing
446. University of Kentucky
447. University of Kentucky College of Dentistry
448. University of Louisville
449. University of Louisville School of Dentistry
450. University of Maryland at Baltimore
451. University of Maryland at Baltimore College of Dental Surgery
452. University of Maryland at Baltimore School of Nursing
453. University of Miami
454. University of Michigan
455. University of Michigan College of Pharmacy
456. University of Michigan Medical School
457. University of Michigan School of Dentistry
458. University of Michigan School of Nursing
459. University of Michigan School of Public Health
460. University of Minnesota
461. University of Mississippi Medical Center
462. University of Mississippi Medical Center School of Dentistry
463. University of Missouri at Kansas City School of Dentistry

464. University of Montana School of Pharmacy and Allied Health Sciences
465. University of Nebraska Medical Center
466. University of Nebraska Medical Center College of Dentistry
467. University of Nevada, Las Vegas School of Dental Medicine
468. University of Nevada, Reno School of Medicine
469. University of North Carolina, Chapel Hill
470. University of North Dakota
471. University of North Texas Health Science Center
472. University of Oklahoma College of Dentistry
473. University of Oklahoma Health Sciences Center
474. University of Oregon
475. University of Pennsylvania School of Dental Medicine
476. University of Pennsylvania School of Medicine
477. University of Pennsylvania School of Nursing
478. University of Pittsburgh Graduate School of Public Health
479. University of Pittsburgh School of Dental Medicine
480. University of Pittsburgh School of Medicine
481. University of Pittsburgh School of Nursing
482. University of Rochester Medical Center
483. University of South Carolina Office of Research and Health Sciences
484. University of South Dakota School of Medicine and Health Sciences
485. University of South Florida
486. University of South Florida College of Nursing
487. University of Southern California
488. University of Tennessee Health Science Center

489. University of Tennessee HSC College of Nursing
490. University of Texas Health Science Center at Houston
491. University of Texas Health Science Center at San Antonio
492. University of Texas M.D. Anderson Cancer Center
493. University of Texas Medical Branch at Galveston School of Medicine
494. University of Texas Southwestern Medical Center at Dallas
495. University of Toledo Academic Health Science Center
496. University of Utah HSC School of Medicine
497. University of Vermont College of Medicine
498. University of Washington
499. University of Wisconsin System
500. University of Wisconsin-Madison
501. Us Too International Prostate Cancer Education and Support Network
502. Van Andel Research Institute
503. Vanderbilt University and Medical Center
504. Virginia Commonwealth University School of Dentistry
505. Virginia Commonwealth University School of Medicine
506. Wake Forest University School of Medicine
507. Washington University in St. Louis
508. West Virginia University Health Sciences Center
509. West Virginia University School of Dentistry
510. Whitehead Institute for Biomedical Research
511. WiCell Research Institution
512. Wisconsin Alumni Research Foundation
513. Wisconsin Association for Biomedical Research and Education
514. Woodruff Health Sciences Center at Emory University
515. X PRIZE Foundation Inc.

516. Yale University School of Medicine
517. Yale University School of Nursing
518. Y-ME National Breast Cancer Organization[62]

What happened to government "of the people, by the people, for the people," as Lincoln put in his immortal Gettysburg Address? Surveys show that more than 70 percent of the American people are in favor of stem cell research using blastocysts leftover from IVF. If our elected officials refuse to vote according to the wishes of the majority of citizens, it is time we voted them out.

Hopefully, the new Congressional team will work from an informed, unbiased, accurate, and truly ethical opinion based upon science rather than upon distorted information provided by the lobbyists of the religious right.

It is wrong that an ideological minority can have so much influence that it can actually block legislative bills in favor of blastocyst stem cell research funding. We must balance that influence with the voices of Americans in favor of research for cure. The squeaky wheel gets the oil, so they say. Maybe it is time for more of us to start squeaking.

Chapter Twelve

POSSIBLE TREATMENTS FROM STEM CELL RESEARCH

Researchers across the globe think there is a good chance of finding treatments for disease through blastocyst stem cell research because they are pluripotent—having both the capacity to become any type of cell and the ability to reproduce more cells while remaining undifferentiated. Supporters of the research say it holds unrivalled promise of new medical treatments for diseases such as Parkinson's disease, diabetes, heart disease, stroke, arthritis, birth defects, cancer, osteoporosis, spinal cord injury, burns, and Alzheimer's disease.

Prominent stem cell biologist Dr. John A. Kessler believes that stem cell biology will revolutionize the practice of medicine:

> *Illnesses such as heart attacks, diabetes, Parkinson's disease, spinal-cord injury, and many others will be treatable. The issue is simply too important to leave to the mercy of uninformed politicians being swayed by a small but vocal group of people with their own agendas.*
>
> *When I was a medical student, I was dismayed to discover how little could be done for patients whose brains or spinal cords*

were injured by trauma or disease. I resolved to devote my career as a neurologist to trying to devise techniques for repairing the damaged nervous system….. However, the extraordinary progress in the field of stem cell biology now makes this a realistic goal. It is truly a joy to think that a lifelong dream of helping neurologically crippled patients may actually come true.[63]

This is a partial list of prestigious organizations supporting stem cell research:

- American Association for the Advancement of Science
- American Diabetes Association
- American Medical Association
- Association of American Medical Colleges
- Christopher Reeve Foundation
- CNS Foundation
- Cure Paralysis Now
- CuresNow
- Juvenile diabetes Research Foundation
- Michael J. Fox Foundation
- Missouri Coalition for Lifesaving Cures and Embryonic Stem Cell Research
- National Health Council
- National MS Society
- Parkinson's Action Network
- The National Coalition for Cancer Research

No one is willing to invest money in something they don't believe will return a benefit (or profit). The results of preliminary animal and human studies using all types of stem cells have been very promising. By pursuing a career in stem cell research, men and women are giving their time and talent to a cause they believe will produce a cure for disease. The fact that private companies are investing millions of dollars into IV-B stem cell research shows that they believe the research will ultimately be financially worthwhile.

The government has appropriated funds for adult stem cell research for years, and we have treatment available that has resulted in cures for many types of cancer. As of 2001, the federal government began to allot funds for a limited range of research on IV-B stem cells created before August 2001. This decision shows that the government must believe stem cell research holds a promise for cures of disease and physical conditions. President Bush acknowledged this fact in his 2006 veto message.

Even with limited funding and restrictions on protocol, there is significant reason to believe that stem cells from blastocysts hold the key to a reproducible source of replacement tissue for human body repair. And, it's not as far away as you might think. Advanced Cell Technology (ACT) raised millions of dollars for stem cell technology by selling convertible debt and by exercising warrants on its stock. The company plans to be ready by the end of next year to request U.S. Food and Drug Administration approval to begin human trials for treatment of macular degeneration.

Aside from those who might win recognition for scientific achievement or receive any monetary benefit are the sick and injured who might be helped by new stem cell therapies resulting from stem cell research. Here are a few stories from patients or family members of patients who have disorders and illnesses that may be helped by stem cell implants.

A 58-year-old paralyzed Vietnam veteran said he hopes progress comes quickly because many paralyzed veterans are praying for treatments.

One of the world's best-known scientists, Stephen Hawking,

suffers from motor-neurone disease (ALS). When Bush vetoed H.R. 810 Hawking said:

> *Banning the use of stem cells from human embryos is the equivalent of opposing the use of donated organs from dead people. The fact that the cells may come from embryos is not an objection because the embryos are going to die anyway. It is morally equivalent to taking a heart transplant from a victim of a car accident.*[64]

Victims of Spinal Cord Injury

Members of the New York State Center of Research Excellence in Spinal Cord Injury conducted a study on rats with Spinal Cord Injury (SCI) and published their findings in the *Journal of Biology*. Stem cell-like cells from the central nervous system, called "embryonic glial restricted precursors cells," were coaxed into differentiating into a specific type of immature astrocytes supportive of nerve fiber growth. These cells were transplanted into cuts in the spinal cord of adult rats that had spinal cord injury. The transplanted cells were marked with dye so the growth could be measured. The study showed that more than 60 percent of the rats' sensory nerve fibers regenerated without scar formation at the injury site. (Scar tissue build-up stabilizes injured central nervous system but will keep stem cell transplants from repairing damage).

Within eight days, approximately two-thirds of the nerve fibers had grown all the way through the injury sites. Within two weeks, the rats were able to walk normally. The rats that received transplants of normal precursor cells that were not transformed into nerve cells had less favorable results. These cells did not suppress scar formation or promote the growth of nerve fibers at the injury site. Four weeks after surgery, the rats that received undifferentiated precursor cells showed little recovery and still had difficulties walking. None of the rats were exhibiting symptoms noting rejection of the cells.

Comparable studies at the University of Louisville showed similar results. These studies show the importance of introducing the right cell types needed for repairing spinal cord injuries, multiple sclerosis, Parkinson's disease, and other nerve disorders. The amazing thing about this research is the cells used on the rats were taken from the tissue of a human nose that controls the ability to smell. The researchers at the University of Louisville report that clinical trials in humans could begin within three to ten years.

Humans with spinal cord injury stand to benefit from treatment and technology derived from all types of stem cell research.

Christopher Reeve

Christopher Reeve was one of the first activists to recognize the potential of stem cell research for the millions of Americans living with paralysis. He was able to communicate that potential to politicians and the public.

"Stem cells have already cured paralysis in animals," Christopher Reeve, the actor known for his role as Superman, said in a commercial he filmed for California's *Yes on Proposition 71* campaign.

In the ad, which was broadcast after his death, he urged voters to "stand up for those who can't."

In a letter to Don C. Reed, Christopher wrote, "One day, Roman and I will stand up from our wheelchairs and walk away from them forever."

Don still believes in that dream. "I intend to see my son walk again one day," he said. "It'll happen. But, only if we elect men and women who care and who can think for themselves."

The Christopher Reeve Foundation (CRF) advocates for expanded scientific inquiry and is the voice of over four million people living with paralysis who could potentially benefit from blastocyst stem cell research.

"This is not a partisan issue," says Maggie Goldberg, spokesperson for the Foundation. "CRF believes in unfettered medical research and supports federal funding and oversight of human embryonic stem cell research."

The goals of CRF were not impacted by the President's veto of H.R 810, but it was a set back. The majority of Americans support IV-B stem cell research and so does the majority of the members of both House and Senate. And, as this book is about to go to print, the House of Representatives and Congress have passed H.R. 3 and Senate Bill 5, respectively—to overturn President Bush's restrictions on IV-B stem cell research. This field of research is changing daily and even faster now that Democrats have control of the House and Senate. Therefore, I will be offering periodic updates on my website www.right2recover.com.

This bill, also known as the Stem Cell Research Enhancement Act of 2007, can make a difference for the millions of Americans living with diseases, injury, and birth conditions who could potentially benefit from stem cell research. Nobel laureates, virtually every major medical and scientific professional association, major research universities and institutions, and affected patient advocacy organizations all support the Stem Cell Research Enhancement Act. These groups have made the bill's passage a top priority.

CRF believes that stem cell research has promise for patients with spinal cord injuries. According to a statement issued by the Foundation in January 2007, IV-B stem cell research looks hopeful for treating spinal cord injuries:

These cells could be the missing links to potentially cure some of the world's most deadly diseases. Stem cell research in spinal cord injury has shown the myelin sheath that covers the spinal cord like telephone cord insulation can actually be re-grown. It could mean that someone who can't even open his or her hand, push a button or hold a pencil could now regain that function. It may sound like a small step but that is huge for someone who is quadriplegic.

Stem cell research is one of the major areas where CRF provides substantial funding, but this is not its only area of research. Not wanting to have all its eggs in one basket, CRF supports many potential avenues for cures. Cures often come from a combination of therapies and, while important, stem cell research is just one of them.

Although help may be years away, people living with paralysis have hope that IV-B research can improve their condition.

Quadriplegia and Paraplegia

Quadriplegia refers to the four limbs (arms and legs) of the body. Approximately 150,000 people in America are quadriplegic—each having varying degrees of function of their arms and legs depending upon the type of spinal injury. Paraplegia is an inability to move the lower body. Like those with spinal cord injury, stem cells offer hope to quadriplegia and paraplegia patients.

Michael Davis's diving accident at age thirteen left him with an incomplete severance of his spinal cord at the cervical level C-4 (neck) region resulting in limited use of his upper extremities. Although he cannot walk, he can use his upper body to do some things for himself. Over the years, he has recovered some wrist flexion and the ability to write, brush his teeth, wash his face, and feed himself. He has quadriplegia. Still, Michael does not call himself handicapped.

Although wheelchair bound, Michael is fortunate enough to be among the 33 percent of the estimated 250,000 persons with spinal cord injury in the U.S. who are able to work a job. He is the executive director of The Independent Living Center of Mobile, Alabama where, for the past two decades, he has managed the day-to-day operations of the center. Its mission is: to foster and promote programs that enable persons with disabilities to attain their maximum level of independence.

Systems change is a major focal point for independent living centers throughout the country. Along with members of his staff, Michael is involved in educating legislators at the local, state, and national levels about the importance of proposed bills, policies, laws, and legislation that affect the rights of persons with disabilities. Serving as the chairman of the Mayor's Advisory Commission for the Disabled in the City of Mobile has positioned Michael to influence the City Council and Mayor about the needs of persons with disabilities and ensure that the "voice" of the disabled community is heard at every level of city government including: employment, transportation, recreation, education, and housing.

In 2005, the Independent Living Center of Mobile sponsored a workshop provided by one of the University of South Alabama's researchers where Michael was enlightened about the possibilities of stem cell technology. He believes this research has remarkable potential to help persons like him who have spinal cord injuries (SCI). He understands that stem cells may have the ability to rebuild most areas of the body as they regenerate and change from one type of cell into another. When introduced intravenously into the brain of a rat, healthy stem cells will immediately seek out injured brain cells and begin producing conditions that stimulate other cells to grow and form new connections among cells. If this transformation helps restore motor function in spinal cord injured rats, surely it can do the same for humans.

Michael has endured many years of pain, and, like most people, he would like to alleviate his suffering. When asked what a cure from stem cell implants would do for him, he replied:

> *I dream of being able to walk again, to feel the warm sand of a beach under my feet, to swim in the Gulf of Mexico, and to cut my own lawn. I would play the keyboard again, shoot baskets with my friends, and finally give my younger brother that long overdue butt kicking I promised him years ago. I think most of all of how I'd love to pick up my wife, whirl her around, lay her gently on our bed, lay beside her and tell her of the wonderful thing God did for me when he brought her my way. While a total cure may be just a theory or hope today, the promise is powerful enough that my dream could very possibly become a reality.*

Michael is able to drive a specially equipped van thanks to computer technology and the miracle of science. He says:

> *Had the world listened to the Uni-bomber and subscribed to his manifesto about the "dangers" of computers, people like me would be hampered from working, voting independently, ambulating with devices, hearing, seeing, or really living. We would not have organ transplants that have added years to the lives of those who suffer with heart, lung, or kidney failure. Our president and a small segment of our population should not impede medical advancements and scientific progress. In a word, I'm all for stem cell research.*

RIGHT TO RECOVER—*Yvonne Perry*

Stroke and Head Injury

Brian Bloodworth is the son of Reverend and Mrs. Dan Bloodworth. Brian made the All-American list after attending an invitational camp in Cincinnati, Ohio. Among those in attendance were Alonzo Morning, Shawn Kemp, and other guys who are now pro basketball players. Brian never knew that he was the fifth best recruit out of the 450 players who were invited to the camp. On August 19, 1987, Brian was riding a steel-wheeled roller while paving the parking lot of a church when he was struck by lightning.

The incident rendered Brian incapacitated. Due to brain damage, he cannot communicate in any way, and he is wholly dependent upon others to care for him. Dan and Carol were heartbroken; not only for their own loss, but for the loss everyone experienced when the world lost the gifts and talents Brian would have offered. Their grief and despair led them to seek cures that might restore their son's health. Desperate to get help in any way possible to improve Brian's condition, the Bloodworth's took their son to the healing ministry of an evangelist who came to town. Brian was strapped in a wheelchair, but, when the family arrived, they couldn't get in the main entrance because the venue was not handicapped accessible. They pushed Brian one block down the street to another hotel that connected with the Convention Center. They used the elevator there, and then maneuvered all the way back to the upper level of the main entrance. The miracle of healing they had hoped for did not take place.

Dan took it upon himself to change the way things worked. He founded The Brian Bloodworth Stroke and Head Injury Research Foundation, Inc. and began studying stem cell research when he heard there was a possibility of healing through IV-B stem cells. His research put him in email and phone contact with

Dr. Evan Snyder, who was then a faculty member in the Neurology Department at Harvard's Beth Israel Deaconess Medical Center in Boston. Dan has sat face-to-face with Senator Frist sharing his Biblical references and medical research information. Regardless of the time and energy Dan and others have spent lobbying to get blastocystic stem cell research approved and funded by our government, President Bush vetoed Stem Cell Research Enhancement Act after it unanimously passed Congress with a strong bi-partisan majority.

Dan is upset with President George W. Bush for vetoing H. R. 810 saying, "He is not a leader of the public or the majority that he says he is. He represents himself to be a Christian believer yet he teaches terror, fear, and his own agenda. The Bible says that God didn't give us a spirit of fear, but of power, love, and of a sound mind. (2 Timothy 1:7). Bush is a deceiver in every way."

Dan will not give up hope for Brian or be discouraged from his efforts to get blastocystic stem cell research funded by the U.S. Government. He is convinced that his son can be helped by therapies resulting from IV-B stem cell research.

Alzheimer's

Alzheimer's is a complex disease most prominent among the elderly. Alzheimer's disease causes the gradual loss of brain cells, resulting in memory loss, disorientation, and ultimately death. The areas of the brain that control memory and thinking skills are affected first, but, as the disease progresses, cells die in other regions of the brain. Eventually, a person with Alzheimer's will need complete care.[65]

Most scientists believe that Alzheimer's disease begins with the buildup of beta amyloid protein in the brain, which may damage the brain years before symptoms appear. Although some existing drug treatments can improve or stabilize symptoms and a great deal of research on new treatments is underway, there is currently no cure for Alzheimer's.

There is great enthusiasm in the scientific community in regard to stem cell research leading to better treatments, or perhaps even a cure for certain diseases. Blastocystic stem cell research offers the most hope in the battle against PD, Type-1 diabetes and spinal cord injury where cell repair can be directed to a defined target. Since the cell damage associated with Alzheimer's disease spreads to large areas of the brain and involves the loss of large numbers and types of the brain's nerve cells, connections, or synapses, the potential of stem cell therapy to correct this widespread destruction is unclear. Newly implanted cells may be able to create new neural connections, but they would not have the lifetime of connections as older cells and would not be able to retain previously stored memories. However, longer-term investigation is needed before any assumptions can be made.

The goal of the Alzheimer's Association is to eradicate the disease through legitimate scientific research that abides by appropriate boundaries for scientific review and ethical guidelines. However, human stem cell research is not a current priority for the Association. Instead, their focus is on understanding the role of amyloid in the brain, risk factors, therapies to slow or stop the progression of the disease, and brain imaging for early diagnosis.

Michael Shelanski is a stem cell researcher and the co-director of the Taub Institute for Research on Alzheimer's disease and the Aging Brain at the Columbia University Medical Center in New York. He believes that while the immediate chances of repairing damage done to the brains of Alzheimer's patients is slim, there may be other therapies for Alzheimer's coming a lot sooner if stem cell research is allowed to expand. Blastocystic stem cell research will at least allow for studies to help identify the molecular errors that underlie Alzheimer's. This discovery would help chemists create drugs to slow, or even reverse, the disease.

Ronald Reagan Family

A high-profile figure and major advocate for stem cell research focusing on treatment for Alzheimer's is Former U.S. First Lady Nancy Reagan. Mrs. Reagan's comments urging the Bush Administration to support IV-B stem cell research add a powerful Republican voice to the debate. With scientists showing Alzheimer's to be the least likely disease to be cured via stem cell therapy, why has Mrs. Reagan become a stem cell activist? Nancy Reagan became interested in stem cells and their theoretical potential for treating Alzheimer's when her husband, former President Ronald Reagan, was suffering with Alzheimer's, but her passion is also stirred by her friendship with Hollywood personalities and moviemakers. Jerry and Janet Zucker, Doug Wick and Lucy Fisher, all have children with diabetes. Together they have drafted blastocystic stem cells into the war on Alzheimer's. They are having an impact even on Republicans and abortion opponents who now agree that blastocystic stem cell research should be funded by the government. Jerry and Janet Zucker contributed more than $50,000 to Proposition 71 to help fund research on blastocyst stem cells. The Zuckers were also one of the three prinicpal proponent families who drafted Proposition 71 and then saw it qualify for the ballot.[66]

Mrs. Reagan is not advocating for stem cell research for Alzheimer's alone. She joined with Michael J. Fox, who suffers from Parkinson's disease, in a fundraiser to raise about $2 million for the Juvenile diabetes Research Foundation. The Juvenile diabetes Research Foundation in turn has contributed $500,000 to the California campaign. As much as Nancy, Ron, and Patti have supported blastocystic stem cell research, adopted son Mike protests against it. Mike Reagan is a board member of the John Douglas French Alzheimer's Foundation. Mike says he's with his dad on stem cell research stating that Ronald Reagan, during his lifetime, opposed the creation of human embryos for the sole purpose of using their stem cells as possible medical cures. I don't know of anyone who is an advocate for creating blastocysts for the sole purpose of research. There are more than enough leftovers in IVF clinics to supply the need. Nevertheless, in an article I found on Cagle Cartoons, Inc., Mike Reagan referred to something his father said in 1983:

> *My administration is dedicated to the preservation of America as a free land and there is no cause more important for preserving that freedom than affirming the transcendent right to life of all human beings, the right without which no other rights have any meaning.*[67]

This does not suggest that Ronald Reagan, Sr. was against blastocystic research. It seems to me, he was stating his pro-life position that all human beings have a right to life. That would mean those who are alive and breathing, not a clump of cells in a laboratory.

There's another quote from Former President Ronald Reagan that says, "While I take inspiration from the past, like most Americans, I live for the future." I believe he would have been proud to support a healthy future for Americans through treatments and therapies derived from stem cells.

RIGHT TO RECOVER—*Yvonne Perry*

Parkinson's Disease

Former Superman actor, Christopher Reeve, was left severely disabled following a riding accident. Former President, Ronald Reagan, suffered with Alzheimer's for ten years before his death. Perhaps some stem cell-derived treatment could have helped them if there had been more time, less government hindrance, and more federal funds for blastocyst stem cell research. While it is too late to help either of these great men, there is hope that others might not have to follow their fate.

Michael J. Fox

Another prominent figure advocating for blastocystic stem cell research is actor Michael J. Fox, who (believe it or not, Rush Limbaugh) suffers from Parkinson's disease. By the way, I am constantly amazed at the ignorance of Rush Limbaugh who said that Fox, being an actor, was either faking his symptoms or was deliberately off his medication in order to exhibit exaggerated symptoms for dramatic effect on TV. Mr. Limbaugh has been known to attack anyone who challenges President Bush and his policies. What is frightening is that there are millions of people who are too lazy, too busy, too whatever, to think for themselves, and they take everything Limbaugh says as the gospel truth. The awkward, involuntary movement Mr. Fox was making during the television commercial is called "Dyskinesia," which is caused from taking Siminet (a common drug given to Parkinson's patients). If Fox hadn't taken his meds, we would have seen tremors, jerking, and shaking that are difficult to imitate. The sad truth is, Fox's condition is really much worse than it appeared in the ad. Worse yet, there is currently no FDA-approved adult stem cell treatment and no cure of any kind for Parkinson's disease.

Not only does Mr. Fox hope to personally benefit from treatment that might be discovered, his concern is also for all those who might be helped by stem cell research. He is doing this by appearing in television commercials and endorsing politicians who support the research. While the veto was not a surprise to Mr. Fox, it still hurt.

CAMR is the nation's leading pro-cures alliance. It is made up of patient organizations, universities, scientific communities, and foundations in favor of research and technologies in regenerative medicine. This includes stem cell research and somatic cell nuclear transfer. CAMR works with elected officials to bring about federal blastocystic stem cell legislation that will move America forward in the fields of science and medicine. Sean Tipton, President of CAMR, says he is thankful for the efforts of Michael J. Fox and the millions of Americans affected with debilitating diseases who are advocating for federal funding of stem cell research.

Mr. Fox has joined forces with some political delegates to further his cause for a cure. Democrat Claire McCaskill, supportive of stem cell research referendum, defeated incumbent Senator Jim Talent who sided with Bush on the veto of H.R. 810. Other supporters of IV-B stem cell research, Rep. Mike Castle (R-DE) and Rep. Diana DeGette (D-CO), as well as Senators Orrin Hatch (R-UT), Ted Kennedy (D-MA), and Dianne Feinstein (D-CA) were re-elected. Mr. Fox also endorsed Tammy Duckworth (D-MD), Senator Ben Cardin, and Governor Jim Doyle. Former Missouri Senator John Danforth (R) became a leader in the fight for stem cell research when his brother died of ALS in 2001. Senator Danforth said:

There are a lot of Republicans who feel strongly that these cells in a Petri dish are the equivalent of a person, and there are other Republicans who feel that these cells in a dish not implanted in a mother are not the equivalent of a person. When you see somebody you love suffer and die from one of these diseases, and medical researchers say this could be the key to finding the cure, then you want the researchers to go forward so other people won't go through the same experience.[68]

Chuck McCann

Chuck McCann is 76 years old and says nature has conspired to control his life in a manner that displeases him. He was diagnosed with Parkinson's in 1984. He was forced into an early retirement in June of 1986, but he refuses to give up on living a full and enjoyable life.

In spite of shaking and sometimes having to use a cane to walk, he continues to bowl three times a week and play doubles tennis one day a week. He fell while playing tennis and is healing during the writing of this book; still he does not give up. Chuck enjoys gardening, playing golf, and walking in the mall. Chuck sculpts in clay; paints pastoral scenes on driftwood, tools, rocks, and feathers; and sells his acrylic creations at local street art fairs. He believes his creativity helps him move past the pain and pity that a lot of senior citizens experience due to aging.

There are treatments available for Parkinson's, and Chuck volunteered to take some experimental prescription drugs in 1986. Not seeing much improvement, his doctor suggested he stop the drugs and take nothing. He stopped all drugs until his doctor died ten years later. Today, Chuck is on Requip to control the shaking produced by Parkinson's disease and his condition is hardly noticeable, and shaking is minimal unless he's under stress or worried about something. If he gets excited, angry, or tired the shaking is worse. At times his left wrist curls and shakes like someone playing a craps table. Drinking from a cup or glass is a problem sometimes as he ends up spilling much of the liquid. Although he cannot write legibly with a pen, he continues to craft creative non-fiction on the computer and participate in a writer's group. Lack of motor control causes him to drool, punch, and kick in his sleep resulting in both him and his wife, Rita, being bruised. At times, he drags his left foot due to a knee problem and uses a motorized chair to help him get up from his frequent naps. The active routine he adheres to is very tiring, but Chuck realizes that if he were to stop he would die.

Mr. McCann has read about stem cell technology, and his family and friends have pointed out articles or research being done. When asked what he thought about having stem cell research to treat his condition he replied, "I don't know if stem cells will help me. I'm 76, and most researchers want younger people to test. I would give it a try, but I don't wish to chase after it."

Taryn Simpson

Taryn Simpson is a published author and a fulltime freelance writer. She has been diagnosed with Young Onset Parkinson's Disease since the age of 40. Here is her story about living with Parkinson's.

One morning I looked at my right hand and noticed that my ring finger was shaking or tremoring by itself. "Oh, it's just nerves....I've been under a lot of stress lately at work and it will settle down once I take a day or two off."

But it didn't. In fact, it was getting worse.

RIGHT TO RECOVER—*Yvonne Perry*

Okay, I'll go see the doctor about it. She'll probably laugh and tell me it is just my nerves. So, I found myself sitting on the examination table and my ring finger was at it again. She looked at it closely and compared it with my other hand. She looked at the fingers next to my shaking ring finger.

"Sure, they're not moving, but it's just nerves, right?"

She frowned as she asked me to do some dexterity exercises. She wrote down a neurologist's name and told me to see him as soon as possible. Then I was concerned because SHE was concerned.

Next thing I knew, I was on the neurologist's exam table. He looked at my shaking finger, and did more dexterity tests and checked my reflexes. He watched me walk down the hallway. He sat on his stool and watched my face for a long period of time. I tried to tell him, "Doc, really....it's just nerves," but he continued his exam. He swiveled around, wrote something in my chart and prescribed a medication.

"Anyone in your family have Parkinson's?" he asked.

I thought for a moment and remembered my great uncle who had it. "Yes."

He looked at me and told me, "It's not your nerves; it's not stress at work. Miss, you have Young Onset Parkinson's Disease. Here are some pamphlets and a prescription for Sinemet. Call me if you have any questions. I will let your doctor know the diagnosis."

I took the pamphlets, the prescription, and walked out of the office on remote control. I made it to my car and sat inside for a few stunned moments. Then I cried.

RIGHT TO RECOVER—*Yvonne Perry*

So what does it feel like? What are some symptoms besides shaking?

In order to help me out here, I called upon a YOPD (Young Onset Parkinson's Disease) friend of mine, who is struggling with it more than I am. Parkinson's disease (PD) affects sleep, causes difficulty in walking, balance, and more.

My symptoms are tremors of the right hand, feeling faint when standing after being seated for awhile, depression, exhaustion, weakness in my legs and hands, loss of smell, falling, balance problems, and restless leg syndrome.

The most aggravating symptom by far is feeling faint upon standing—that, and actually falling. People think I am drunk when this happens. It also hurts when I fall. I guess it's a blessing for all the padding that I have back there!

My Fellow PDer's symptoms include tremors all over his body, problems with walking and sleeping, balance, exhaustion, depression, and general weakness in his body. His most aggravating symptom is difficulty with walking and functioning normally i.e.: problems with buttoning shirts, holding a coffee cup without spilling the contents, walking without "freezing in place" while waiting for his feet to cooperate with his brain, and physical exhaustion.

Is PD fatal? I suppose it can be, as it can cause choking on saliva or food, etc. But, for the most part, it's just a pain in the butt. Literally, in my case.

For the most part, I'm doing pretty well. My meds keep my symptoms in check (except the falling, but oh well). I have a sense of humor about it and proudly wear my shirt that reads,

RIGHT TO RECOVER—*Yvonne Perry*

"I'm Not Getting Jiggy with it. I Have Parkinson's" to my doctor
appointments. It makes everyone laugh...including ME.

Taryn brought up an interesting point when I asked her if
she thought an embryo is actually being killed through stem cell
research. She does not believe an embryo is being killed, but she
reminded me that some people have the incorrect notion that stem
cells used for IV-B stem cell research are fertilized inside a woman's
body as part of the beginning stages of life, and then removed for
research purposes. I was dumbfounded! I didn't know anyone was
that ignorant about the topic! No wonder people think blastocyst
stem cell research is equal to abortion. Surely, if you've read this far
in my book, you know that *"in vitro"* means that the egg and sperm
are united in a lab dish outside the body; and you understand that
a blastocyst requires nourishment and "instructions" from the
mother's body in order to reach subsequent stages of growth. Stem
cells derived from the inner cell mass of a blastocyst cannot give
rise to a placenta. Therefore, a human being could not possibly
develop from the stem cell lines created from the inner cells of an
IV-B. Creating new stem cell lines through SCNT does not in any
way kill an embryo because there is no embryo—only cells. You
would have to implant the entire blastocyst into the womb in order
to have an embryo.

Ms. Simpson says there is no doubt that researchers will one
day find a cure for Parkinson's disease:

> PD is a disease that involves the inability of the brain
> to produce certain chemicals (dopamine) at normal levels. This
> chemical regulates libido (or depression), movement, etc. If a
> specifically cultured stem cell were transplanted, it would regenerate
> automatically and replace the malfunctioning brain cells. Spinal

cord injuries, Muscular Dystrophy, and other brain-related illnesses would reap the same results…either increased movement or being able to move as normally as anyone else.

Taryn would be willing to try a cure derived from stem cell research but says that she will not be first in line because that place of honor should go to others who are suffering much worse than her. She would like to see those most seriously afflicted with this disease receive treatment first. Perhaps there could be a 1-5 rating scale used by neurologists. Taryn says her condition would only be a one or two, but Michael J. Fox and Muhammad Ali should receive treatment first since they are about a five on the scale.

Diabetes

Islet cells control insulin production in the pancreas. This production is disrupted in people having diabetes. A logical cure would be to restore insulin-producing islet cells so they function normally. This can occur either through islet cell transplantation or through production of cells to restore the insulin secreting function. Some clinical trials on humans have been done by injecting patients with pancreatic islet cells derived from cadavers (corpses). Due to the need to administer anti-rejection medications which are harsh on the insulin-producing islet cells, less than eight percent of islet cell transplants are successful.

As you know from earlier in this book, adult stem cells do not have the same capacity as those obtained from blastocysts. Adult stem cells are differentiated. For example, heart stem cells are predisposed to become heart cells and not insulin-producing islet cells or other tissues. Because blastocyst stem cells are primordial cells able to develop into any type of cell or tissue, it may be possible to genetically alter them so they are not susceptible to an immune attack. Blastocyst stem cells will be ideal for treating diabetes provided scientists are able to direct their development into insulin-producing islet cells.

The Juvenile diabetes Research Foundation encourages the pursuit of blastocyst stem cell research within the framework of appropriate scientific and ethical safeguards. Since stem cells from fetal tissue are eligible for federal funding and are not banned by government, they are the primary source of stem cells used for diabetes research. While stem cell research is at a very early stage, it seems to offer great promise for discovery of a cure for diabetes.

Heart Patients

According to the National Institutes of Health, one percent of all newborns born worldwide each year have heart problems. Heart defects are the leading cause of first year infant death in the United States. Many heart valve defects can be detected with ultrasound tests during pregnancy at about twenty weeks of gestation.

Amniotic fluid surrounds and cushions developing embryos in the uterus. The fluid can be obtained through a needle inserted into the womb of a pregnant woman. Swiss scientists isolated fetal stem cells from amniotic fluid, cultured the cells in a lab dish, and then placed them on a mold shaped like a small hollow plastic ink pen. Within six weeks the scientist had grown twelve human heart valves. The purpose for the experiment is to learn more about prenatal fabrication replacement parts. Should the baby be born with a defective heart valve, there would be a valve more durable and effective than an artificial or donated valve waiting to be implanted. Since artificial valves are prone to blood clots, patients receiving them must take anti-clotting drugs for life. Valves from human or animal donors can deteriorate and may require repeated open-heart surgeries to replace them—especially in children whose bodies are still growing when the valve isn't. Lab-grown valves should avoid both these problems, and it stands to reason that the risk of rejection would be minimized since the valves were derived from the donor's own stem cells. Now you understand the importance of collecting and storing fetal cord blood and fluid. By the time your baby is old enough to need replacement parts, the technology to grow the parts from the cells you put "on ice" at birth may be available to save his or her life.

Lab tests showed the Swiss valves appeared to function normally. However, these valves will not be placed into a human just yet. The next step is to see if they work in an animal. Dr. Simon Hoerstrup, a University of Zurich scientist says a two-year experiment with a sheep is under way.

After showing a video clip of beating heart cells derived from blastocyst stem cells, Dr. Kessler said, "I think it's absolutely impossible not to get excited when you see the possibilities of ultimately regenerating the heart with stem cells."

Another exciting announcement coming from two separate groups of U.S. scientists at Harvard is the discovery of "cardiac master cells" that are able to differentiate into cardiac muscle, smooth muscle, or endothelial cells. This research, using blastocyst stem cells from mice, gives hope that therapies may be developed to help human heart attack victims and patients with heart disease. Naturally, the next step is to try to coax human blastocyst stem cells to develop into the kind of cells the researchers identified in mice. The breakthrough here is a better understanding of how to guide blastocystic stem cells to generate specific tissues. This understanding will hopefully shed light on abnormal cell growth and could help treat or even prevent birth defects and cancer. Stem cells could also be used for testing pharmaceutical products on specific cell types, which would aid in the development of drug therapies.

Neurodegenerative Childhood Diseases

Dr. Evan Snyder is both a pediatrician and a lab researcher. He is highly sought after by support and advocacy groups. Snyder's research on Ataxia-Telangiectasia (A-T) is partially funded by the Florida-based A-T Children's Project founded by Brad Margus who has two sons increasingly disabled by A-T. Through these and other private funds, Dr. Snyder is able to bypass the federal system of research grants to focus on rare diseases such as Tay-Sachs, Gaucher, leukodystrophy, Sandhoff, and other neurodegenerative diseases.

A-T is a neurodegenerative childhood disease beginning at a young age that affects the nervous system and other body systems. A-T is marked by a progressive lack of muscle control, which makes it difficult to balance, walk, speak, or swallow. Other symptoms include spider veins, stunted growth, recurring respiratory infections, bronchitis, pneumonia, and immune suppression. A-T victims are highly susceptible to cancer.

Bringing her two children with her, a woman who had heard about the A-T Children's Project came to visit Dr. Snyder. Her little girl had early signs of A-T.

"Do you think you can help her before she gets worse?" the mother asked.

Dr. Snyder says that away from his word processor, slides, or audience of scientists, he gets frightened when he actually meets patients:

RIGHT TO RECOVER—*Yvonne Perry*

There's this combination of both exhilaration and absolute dire panic. The exhilaration is the thought that maybe, maybe I do have in my power the ability to help this kid so that this kid will never develop the symptoms that I know happens with kids with A-T. Then the panic sets in and says "but what if you can't do it." And then the exhilaration comes back and says, "Well, you've got to do it."[69]

Dr. Snyder's research uses human stem cells as an enzyme-replacement tool for children affected by lysosomal storage disorders. A normal brain is able to produce the enzymes that break down unneeded molecules in the cells. A brain with lysosomal storage disorder is unable to produce these important enzymes. When the molecular "garbage" builds to toxic levels within brain cells, normal brain cell function is impaired and ultimately causes brain cell death. Dr. Snyder's experiment with animals modeling the disease will examine the ability of transplanted human brain stem cells to reverse Sandhoff symptoms. He believes transplanted stem cells have the ability to supply missing enzymes, but he will also co-administer drugs that reduce the toxic level of molecular build-up in the Sandhoff-affected brain.

Children's Neurobiological Solutions Foundation (CNS) is a parent-driven non-profit organization fostering the development of true brain repair therapies for special-needs children. Their mission is to expedite the creation of effective treatments and therapies for children having neurodevelopmental abnormalities, injuries to the nervous system, and related neurological problems. CNS also informs families and health care providers with user-friendly access to state-of-the-art information and education to support their decision-making processes. CNS and the A-T Children's Project are also helping to fund Steve Goldman, M.D.,

Ph.D, of the University of Rochester. Dr. Goldman, who will be conducting studies as he prepares for a clinical trial, hopes to be able to repair severe pediatric neurological brain disorders such as Pelizaeus-Merzbacher Disease, Krabbe's Disease, and Tay-Sachs Disease.

The purpose of Dr. Goldman's project, "Perinatal Implantation of Human Glial Progenitor Cells as a Treatment Strategy for Childhood Myelin Disorders," is to analyze specific brain cells, known as oligodendrocyte progenitor cells (OPCs) and their potential to treat myelin disorders in children. The myelin sheath surrounds cells and helps send messages between cells. When the myelin sheath does not form properly, or is lost, brain and spinal function is severely inhibited. Dr. Goldman will begin his research by treating congenital myelin deficiency in mice.

In collaboration with the A-T Children's Project, Children's Neurobiological Solutions Foundation (CNS) awarded research funds to Dr. Evan Snyder, Professor and Director of The Burnham Institute's Stem Cells and Regeneration Program, to investigate the potential use of the brain stem cells as a therapeutic vehicle for Sandhoff Disease.

Immune Deficiencies

An immune deficiency disease occurs when one or more parts of the immune system are missing. These diseases can be inherited, acquired through infections or other illness, or induced as a side effect of drug treatment. Acquired immunodeficiency disease (AIDS) is the most well known, but there are many inherited immunodeficiency diseases which are less common.

The human body has two major types of immunity: antibody-mediated and cell-mediated immunity. Bone marrow stem cells produce pathways to both types of immunity. B cells that produce different antibodies targeted to specific invaders are generated in the lymph nodes and spleen; T cells that directly attack their targets are generated in the thymus gland. Bone marrow transplants have been used to successfully treat children with a diverse group of inherited immune disorders known as chronic granulomatous disease (CGD). CGD shows a defect in an enzyme (*phox*) used by white blood cells to generate the hydrogen peroxide needed to kill bacteria and fungi. This renders the immune system unable to fight off pathogens that cause serious illness. By inserting a correct form of the *phox* gene into precursor immune stem cells from cord blood and transfusing the cells back into a patient, researchers at the National Institute of Allergy and Infectious Diseases (NIAID) devised a gene therapy for CGD.

Arthritis

Rheumatoid arthritis (RA) is a chronic illness characterized by pain, stiffness, inflammation, and redness at the joints, which leads to a loss of movement or function. People with RA may have difficulty grasping a fork, combing hair, or buttoning a shirt. Fatigue, flu-like symptoms (including a low-grade fever), nodules or lumps under the skin, muscle pain, loss of appetite, depression, anemia, weight loss, and muscle pain also accompany the illness.

Arthritis is progressive, and usually begins in the small joints in the fingers, hands, and wrists. However, the illness is systemic, which means it can also affect organs and tissues throughout the body. In later stages the growth of cells in the tissue or lining of the joints releases enzymes that eat away the bone and cartilage. While aggressive treatment in early stages can limit joint damage, there is no cure for RA.

RIGHT TO RECOVER—*Yvonne Perry*

There are many related auto-immune disorders: juvenile rheumatoid arthritis, lupus, rheumatoid arthritis and scleroderma. Their cause may be related to exposure to antigens, which causes a faulty immune system. Therefore, people with RA are more susceptible to infection. Others say that RA is related to aberrant T cell, B cell, and macrophage function. Recent studies may indicate that RA isn't one disease but possibly several different diseases sharing common symptoms.

Researchers in Europe, Australia, and the United States have used bone marrow stem cell transplants to treat several forms of arthritis. This is a risky, investigational procedure that temporarily leaves the patient without an immune system for a while. Therefore, the procedure is only used on patients with severe, life-threatening arthritis who have not responded to standard therapy. The Arthritis Foundation says that the transplants done to date in people with arthritis have only involved bone marrow cells taken from the person with arthritis.

Since RA patients have a faulty immune system, the logic is to remove stem cells from the bone marrow, give high doses of chemotherapy to kill any remaining defective cells, and reintroduce a new, healthy immune system through stem cell transplant. Doctors at Leeds General Infirmary's rheumatology department involved in a two-year study on stem cell transplantation have treated six patients. All but one patient has relapsed. The new immune system is failing like the old one did because bone marrow transplants do not correct the essential fault within the body. The good news is that the five who relapsed are now responding much better to drug therapies that previously had failed to help them.

RIGHT TO RECOVER—*Yvonne Perry*

Multiple Sclerosis

The cause of multiple sclerosis (MS) is not known, but it is an auto-immune disease that triggers the body's immune system to attack and destroy its own nervous system—particularly myelin. Myelin is the fatty coating that insulates nerve cells in the central nervous system and enables messages to be sent. Stripped of myelin (much like electric wires whose insulation has been partially removed), nerve cells malfunction and cause reduced vision, loss of balance, progressive weakness, memory loss, and localized paralysis.

Existing drug treatments for MS suppress the immune attack but only temporarily halt the progression of the disease rather than reversing the symptoms. According to a team study at Yale University, it is possible to use stem cells extracted from a patient's bone marrow to repair the nerve cell damage caused by MS. Dr. Jeffery Kocsis, associate director of the Neuroscience and Regeneration Research Center of Yale University, said, "The beauty of the potential use of bone marrow is you don't have to go into the brain to remove nerve (stem) cells." Kocsis and his team transplanted stem cells from adult bone marrow into rats. The results show substantial regrowth of important nerve cells. The research is still in early stages, but the first safety testing in humans could begin within one year.

A team led by Bruce Brew at Saint Vincent's Hospital in Sydney, Australia confirmed the results of the experiment on mice. The team found that the stem cells were able to find areas of brain damage and differentiate into cells that manufacture myelin (oligodendrocytes). Brew hopes the new oligodendrocytes will be capable of repairing myelin enough to sufficiently reduce symptoms. He also hopes his stem cell technique could be used to tackle other illnesses such as meningitis and encephalitis.

Due to the lack of controversy over umbilical cord stem cell therapy, the U.S. is already beginning to use cord blood therapies.

Autism

Autism is a complex disorder of brain function that manifests before the age of three. Autistic children have problems with social interaction, communication, imagination, and behavior. Autistic characteristics may persist into adulthood. While the cause for autism is unknown, a lack of blood flow in both the left and right temporal lobes has been seen in children with primary autism. The right superior temporal area related to processing social, sensory, and emotional information is reduced in autistic children.

Current treatment involves nutritional and antioxidant therapies, elimination of heavy metal toxicity and bacterial overgrowth, and the repair of brain lesions. Blood stem cells from umbilical cord blood can help in cases that show a lack of blood flow, or a diminished volume of glial cells (white matter), in the brain. These cells have the ability to promote the growth of new blood vessels, glial cells, and neural progenitor cells. Eight children diagnosed with autism received a cord blood stem cell infusion in Mexico. The parents report some improvement in eye contact and social interaction.

Osteoporosis

Osteoporosis is a degenerative bone disease that causes bones to become fragile and more likely to break. Osteoporosis or "porous bone," is characterized by a decrease in bone density due to the loss of calcium and collagen. Approximately 55 percent of Americans aged 50 years and older have the disease; most are women. As our population ages, the number of people needing treatment for age-related bone loss increases. Costs for hospitals and nursing home cares for osteoporotic and associated fractures was $17 billion in 2001.

A group of researchers from The Skaggs Institute for Chemical Biology at The Scripps Research Institute and from the Genomics Institute of the Novartis Research Foundation (GNF) have reported how a small synthetic molecule called "purmorphamine" causes multipotent mesenchymal progenitor cells to differentiate into adult bone cells. By using high-density oligonucleotide microarrays to monitor the stem cells' gene behavior following treatment with purmorphamine, Doctors Wu, Ding, Schultz, and their teams identified a cluster of genes that "notified" other cells to produce a type of protein called hedgehog. The hedgehog protein activates a number of genes that encourage proliferation and differentiation for the cell to transform into an osteocyte. Purmorphamine is hoped to have significant clinical value for treating the bone-weakening disease osteoporosis.

If you were suffering from a disease and felt sure there was a remedy waiting to be discovered, wouldn't you want science to move forward so you and others could benefit from it? I don't understand why anyone would want to withhold support for research that might give way to treatment for diseases and injuries. We all stand to benefit from stem cell research. Every type of stem cell is important because of the variety of abilities each has. Different technologies, drugs and therapies derived from stem cell research will one day be common place. The research must go on unhindered.

Chapter Thirteen

TURNING THE TIDES TOWARD THE RIGHT TO RECOVER

I've heard it said many times that it takes an entire village to raise a child. In other words, it is the responsibility of every citizen to look out for the best interests of the entire community. In any way we can, we should try our best to relieve the suffering and pain of as many people as possible.

We are global citizens whether we like it or not. Our neighbor is not just the person living next door. Every human on the planet is our neighbor, and we are told by the Masters to love our neighbor in the same manner we love ourselves. In most cases, biomedical researchers are motivated to help find cures and bring good health to people and the planet. It is our responsibility to join in the effort and do our part.

If, after reading this book, you are still opposed to blastocyst stem cell research and are part of the hindrance that is withholding funds for research, then let me ask you this: If you or a loved one ever need treatment for Alzheimer's, Parkinson's disease, heart disease, spinal cord injury, or another illness or injury, would you accept treatment or therapies derived from human blastocystic stem cell research? If it goes against your morals now, would you change your beliefs rather than let your loved one die when there's help available—help that you tried to prevent others from receiving? I doubt you would let your severely burned daughter die if she could live by having her own skin cells cloned using a stem cell from a blastocyst in a laboratory. You probably wouldn't care then if a blastocyst or an embryo had been destroyed in the process. If you or your loved one needed a heart transplant today, our present technology means that the donor has died. There's no moral issue or guilt to be associated with organ donation, nor should there be, so why continue to hold a non-supportive view of research that might possibly supply new organs and tissues without anyone having to die? Why not change your position now before you or your loved one needs a treatment derived from blastocyst stem cells?

For those who still think blastocyst stem cell research is equal to taking a life, consider this: If one human blastocyst can generate a new line of cells that could help an unlimited number of people, wouldn't it be worth the sacrifice of that one blastocyst? Especially since the alternative is to put them in a bio trash bag—especially when remaining cells of the blastocyst could still be implanted into a womb to produce a healthy fetus? How can this even be considered evil? To allow healthy cells to be thrown away rather than being used to cure disease is merciless!

People, including **ministers**, seem to forget our earthly flesh is only temporal and we **are** spirit having an experience in human form. We wear a suit of flesh during our time on earth but many times this flesh becomes our focus instead of our spirit. We fight to preserve the body and ego instead of concentrating on developing the spirit.

RIGHT TO RECOVER—*Yvonne Perry*

Energy cannot be destroyed, only rearranged. The soul is immortal and does not die when the body does. Life is energy; energy is not destroyed in death, it is transformed into a different type of life. If a blastocyst is pulled apart and put into separate Petri dishes, it doesn't die. It continues to create more life! Biologists simply want to be able to control the form of life it takes in the lab. They are attempting to coax the life force in those cells into creating new cells, nerves, tissues, and possibly organs that can continue to create life inside a living human being.

We live in a give-and-take world, and it requires both sacrifice and compromise to live in harmony with one another. When our country is at war, innocent people are sacrificed to protect our citizens. Regardless of the fact that many people are opposed to the war in Iraq and cry out against it, our government still sends troops overseas to wage battle in a war that cannot be won. Even the government agrees with the philosophy of having one person make a sacrifice for the good of many. Officials may elect to take your land whether you like it or not, if it can be shown that having a new highway on your property would benefit the majority of people in the area. Blastocyst stem cell research is for the good of all humankind.

Conception begins when the blastocyst implants itself into the lining of the uterus. Blastocysts are NOT babies, they are NOT fetuses; they can't truly be called embryos unless they have implanted and are drawing nourishment from a mother. Those abandoned leftovers from *in vitro* procedures will never be implanted into a human womb. A blastocyst is a cluster of cells and is not even an organism. These tiny cells don't think, breathe or have consciousness, yet they could make some dramatic changes for millions of suffering humans who do.

RIGHT TO RECOVER—*Yvonne Perry*

There are scientific and logical reasons why an embryo is NOT being created *or* destroyed in a laboratory:

1. There are only sperm, ova, zygotes, and blastocysts in an *in vitro* lab. A blastocyst is not able to become an embryo in the lab.
2. Embryos form inside a woman's uterus after implantation and conception have occurred.
3. An embryo is a product of a pregnancy, not of a scientific joining of two cells. Pregnancy can only occur in a uterus.
4. An *in vitro* blastocyst from which a stem cell has been removed is still able to be implanted in a uterus and brought to term. No destruction is necessary.

People are desperate for a cure or any help to alleviate their suffering. Dr. Keirstead said he has had people call him and say, "I'm about to commit suicide, do you have anything to stop me?"

People need to know how close scientists are to making viable healing therapies through the miraculous and untapped potential of IV-B stem cell research. This potential will only be discovered through research, and that research will be conducted much quicker when more funds are available. We don't need to slow down our research progress; we need to carefully use stem cells to create a better life for everyone.

If human IV-B stem cell research were publicly funded today, it would still need to be done in a controlled environment with ethical standards and with social investigators from protective committees providing good oversight. Since there are so many unknowns about this technology, we don't know what to expect. We should start with larger animals such as primates, which are much more similar to a human than a rat.

Dr. Gerald Fischbach, director of the National Institute of Neurological Disorders and Stroke, has a positive outlook on the future of stem cell research:

> *Stem cell biology is enormously exciting right now and holds promise for really novel therapies - not just symptomatic therapies, but maybe cures. Before the decade is out, there will be some therapeutic benefits from treating disease with neural stem cells. Parkinson's disease, caused by the death of brain cells in a certain region, might be one of the first targets for stem cell treatment; another is Lou Gehrig's disease, or amyotrophic lateral sclerosis, because it kills so quickly and there's no treatment.*[71]

Ignorance is Not Bliss!

The same questions being asked today were raised with *in vitro* fertilization and have historically been raised with numerous scientific processes that are currently accepted as routine, such as organ transplantation. Today, pacemakers and organ transplants are common medical tools and procedures. Implants derived from adult or cord blood stem cells are used to treat cancer. If you asked an average American family of the 1950s about a new device that could be implanted into the heart to make sure it didn't stop beating, they would have either laughed at you or thought you were trying to play God. Penicillin was the result of fifteen years of research, yet who among us now has not benefited from it? Stem cell technology might not cure the ill and maimed today, but those of the future will definitely benefit from the therapies and pharmaceuticals it will render.

Some of the most important advances in science were opposed due to moral issues surrounding it. DNA and heart transplants were initially opposed on moral grounds. Today, the science has been used to save millions of lives. *In vitro* fertilization was highly controversial when it was introduced in the 1970s, but today it is an accepted solution for millions facing infertility. The well-organized and well-funded minority groups that oppose blastocyst stem cell research are the same groups that opposed organ transplantation, blood transfusions, and other scientific advances that are now everyday medicine. It's normal for humans to balk at change and criticize what they don't understand—especially if a religious or political leader tells them it is unethical or unfeasible.

Think back about thirty years, when receiving a diagnosis of cancer meant you were going to die. There was no cure and very little treatment was proven successful. Federally funded research using cord blood, bone marrow, and adult stem cells has not been halted by moral or religious opposition. As a result, this technology has fostered the growth of a biotech industry that has created drugs for dozens of diseases, not to mention that it also creates jobs and billions of dollars in annual revenues. Just think of the costs associated with medical care to treat illness in the U.S. A cure that would allow people to recover would be much better than a temporary bandage. Without public funding, medical advances in life-saving therapies such as blood transfusion, cancer treatment, and organ transplantation would not have occurred.

We don't have proof that blastocyst stem cells will vastly improve our quality of life. Scientists have not had the opportunity to do the research on a wide scale. However, we have no reason to believe that these cells won't make some wonderful changes either. In fact, research using IV-B stem cells has just as much promise as adult and cord blood stem cells that have differentiated and established themselves as a certain type of cell. If research on IV-

RIGHT TO RECOVER—*Yvonne Perry*

B stem cells were to have the same freedom and funding as adult stem cell research, I can only imagine the results. Literally millions of people might have their lives transformed and their suffering cured if the promise of stem cell research were realized. Perhaps the lame would walk again, the blind would see, and the deaf would hear again. Who knows? Didn't Jesus say that we would do even greater works than he did? This new age of miracles could be the Second Coming of Christ!

If Jesus of Nazareth really did perform miracles and was able to raise the dead almost 2,000 years before defibrillators, he certainly wouldn't condemn us for following his example with medical miracles of our own. God gives us our skills, abilities, and talents to accomplish great the things. This includes medical breakthroughs that help humanity. It's up to us to use these gifts rather than try to prevent them from being shared with others.

To think that a life has been taken by using fertilized eggs for research has to be one of the biggest and most ignorant of all assumptions. One day, this resistance to blastocyst stem cell research will be thought of as an insane waste of time as we look back upon it from the future. We will wonder why we allowed our pro-war President to get away with vetoing a bill that could have provided federal funding for research that has such potential to cure disease—especially while spending billions of dollars on a war that takes the lives of innocent people. We will question the sanity of those who were more concerned with the fate of a 36- to 48-hour-old clump of cells than they were with curing those who had been suffering for decades. We will wonder why a small minority of outspoken citizens of our society, blinded by what they perceived as a religious or moral issue, were allowed to delay possible cures for a number of injuries and medical conditions.

RIGHT TO RECOVER—Yvonne Perry

Relieving Suffering: A Right to Recover

Cells are located throughout our bodies, but they each have different functions. Just as your liver cannot perform the same tasks as your heart, adult stem cells, cord blood, and amniotic stem cells cannot do the same things as blastocyst stem cells. Like a young child, totipotent and pluripotent stem cells possess the ability to become anything they want to be when they grow up. We need to explore all the possibilities without limiting our scope of funding to exclude blastocysts.

Patients are different with respect to how they respond to treatments. What works for one person doesn't necessarily help another person. When it comes to finding a cure, one size never fits all. That is why I am advocating research for all types of stem cell research, not only that done with blastocysts.

Even though it could take a decade or more to develop useful therapies, blastocystic stem cell research holds enormous promise. Therefore, it is important to explore all types: adult stem cells, the cells found in amniotic fluid, cord blood, and the most versatile of all, those derived from blastocysts. Regardless of whether the therapies come from adult stem cells, cord blood, amniotic fluid, or IV-B research, all of humanity stands to profit from stem cell treatment and technology. Whether it comes from the U.S. or another country, the cure for Alzheimer's, Parkinson's, heart disease, spinal cord injury, diabetes, or other illness or injuries is within reach.

Regardless of what right-wingers say or what the government will fund, there is proof that blastocyst stem cell research offers a key to treatment and technology that our forefathers would have thought impossible. In this book we have discussed injuries and diseases being positively affected by stem cell technology. Many more may yet be discovered, but here are a few:

1. Alzheimer's disease
2. Amyotrophic Lateral Sclerosis (ALS) Lou Gehrig's disease
3. Arthritis
4. Autism
5. Birth defects
6. Blindness
7. Blood products
8. Burns
9. Cancer
10. Cerebral Palsy
11. Corneal stem cell transplants
12. Diabetes
13. Heart disease stroke
14. Immune Deficiencies
15. Lou Gehrig's Disease
16. Multiple Sclerosis
17. Nervous system
18. Neurodegenerative brain illnesses
19. Osteoporosis
20. Paraplegia
21. Parkinson's disease
22. Quadriplegia
23. Renal failure
24. Spinal Cord Injury
25. Stroke
26. Traumatic Brain Injury.

RIGHT TO RECOVER—*Yvonne Perry*

In addition to the cures that may be found, there are many economic reasons the research should be funded. Many programs in public schools that meet the needs of students requiring special care are funded by our tax dollars. If a permanent treatment for childhood diseases was found, the money being used to fund these special programs could be used for more research to cure even more illnesses. Think of the out-of-pocket costs a patient with quadriplegia or Parkinson's would save if they didn't need a full-time caregiver or special equipment. Not only is there a personal benefit to patients, curing illnesses clearly provides a benefit to all of society. Insurance rates would decrease if diseases were curable. All this money would flow back into the economy.

If we sit in fear, holding to unfounded mental strongholds and do nothing to stop our government from taking away our rights, we will become slaves to a dictator-ruled government. We need leaders who respect the power of their position. Robert Kennedy once said, "The problem of power is how to achieve its responsible use rather than its irresponsible and indulgent use - of how to get men of power to live *for* the public rather than *off* the public."

Like an unsuspecting frog in a pot of water that is slowly reaching boiling point, U.S. citizens have allowed the government to take more and more of our freedom secured by the Bill of Rights. A minority of religion–crazed citizens are controlling the thermostat through their lobbying and elected term in office. It's time to stand up to government and vote against bills and amendments that take away the one thing our founding fathers did have in common—freedom of religion and separation of Church and State.

End the War

History shows that religious ideological wars in America are not quickly or easily resolved. In that respect, I doubt there is a way to truly "win" the political and religious wars over stem cell research. I do hope this book will at least help circumvent the hostility on both sides of the issues. You can remain a conservative, Christian, a pro-life advocate, Republican, and still support blastocyst stem cell research. By supporting all types of stem cell research there is a better chance for cures for more types of illnesses. It's time to lay down our religious and political weapons and work together for the benefit of all citizens.

War and fighting does not bring peace to any situation. Just look at the war in Iraq. It continues to escalate, people continue to lose their lives and no resolution is in sight. As one who embraces metaphysical concepts, I believe that the power of thought is magnified by numbers. The more people we have fighting and producing negativity and ill-will, the more that mindset will grow. And, the more people we have thinking thoughts of peace and sending love (which casts out fear) and light (which helps us see Divine will), the more peace has a chance to grow. It's like the tuning fork effect that has been noticed by some vibrational scientists. If you strike a higher frequency tuning fork at the same time as other lower frequency tuning forks, the lower ones will automatically raise their frequencies to match the vibration of the higher pitched tuning fork.

Einstein once said, "The religion of the future will be a cosmic religion. It should transcend a personal God and avoid dogmas and theology. Covering both natural and spiritual, it should be based on a religious sense arising from the experience of all things, natural and spiritual and a meaningful unity."

RIGHT TO RECOVER—*Yvonne Perry*

In addition to writing this book, I have also asked ascended masters Jesus Christ, Krishna, Horus, Mother Mary, Quan Yin, Isis, the Bodhisattvas, the Buddhas, and other loving, higher vibrational energies and deities to gently remind all of our elected officials that we are one in Spirit and that we all want what is best for humanity. Each time I feel frustrated about the stem cell battle, I send love and light to the collective consciousness of humanity, the Senate and President Bush. If we are in agreement that God/Goddess's highest and best be done regarding all types of stem cell research, I think it would be a more enlightened approach that might yield miraculous results.

I am praying for a cure for all types of disease and conditions and it doesn't matter to me what research method brings it forward. Even though I've published a book that exposes the truth and lies I've discovered in my research, my motive is not to cause more conflict. My hope is to bring peace to the issue and provide hope to those who suffer. Why not join me in this peaceful effort by simply agreeing in thought or verbal prayer that whatever is best for humanity will be manifest in the decision of our political and religious leaders? It's worth a try, isn't it?

Ways You Can Help

Stem cell biology holds such promise that I consider *in vitro* assisted stem cell research a gift to humanity. Now is the time to begin our efforts to sway public opinion toward the approval of research funds for this important medical breakthrough.

1. Show that you know the difference between a blastocyst and an embryo. Stop referring to blastocyst stem cell research by a term that infers that a life is being taken by research.

2. Contribute corporate donations to not-for-profit biotech companies that support blastocyst stem cell research. These donations are tax deductible. Lottery winners might consider giving a portion of their winnings to research centers or charities that push for legislation to fund all types of stem cell research.
3. Write your Senators and State Legislators asking for their support for federal funding of all types of stem cell research.
4. Share with others what you have learned in this book. I plan to share the profits from the sales of this book with deserving stem cell research centers around the country.
5. Vote for a candidate who supports funding for stem cell research on human blastocysts.
6. Learn more about stem cell research at www.right2recover. com.
7. Focus on what is best for humanity and pray for the well-being of your global neighbors and loved ones.

With recent advancements in biotechnology, it is criminal not to support research that has the potential to benefit those who suffer from injury and disease, or who need organ and tissue replacement. Hopefully, you will support all types of stem cell research and urge our government to separate fact from fiction. By allowing scientists and doctors to explore blastocyst stem cell technology on humans, we are very likely to find a cure for SCI, Alzheimer's, heart disease, Parkinson's, diabetes, cancer, and other illnesses. Just think of all the people you know who would benefit.

Perhaps this book has made you reconsider your religious belief systems. Maybe it has spurred you to take action to become involved in politics. Whatever the result, I trust are all willing to work together to make our world a healthier place.

We all have the *RIGHT TO RECOVER!*

APPENDIX - Chapter Notes

Chapter One

1. Faden, Ruth R. and John D. Gearhart. "Facts on Stem Cells." 23 August 2004. Accessed 10 January 2007. <http://www.washingtonpost.com/wp-dyn/articles/A25071-2004Aug22.html>.

Chapter Two

2. "Definition of Organism." Yahoo Education. Accessed 11 March 2007. <http://education.yahoo.com/reference/dictionary/entry/organism>.

3. "Glossary of Selected Terms." Science and Technology/Engineering Curriculum Framework. Accessed 11 March 2007. <http://www.doe.mass.edu/frameworks/scitech/2001/resources/glossary.html>.

4. "Organism." Wikipedia. Accessed 11 March 2007. <http://en.wikipedia.org/wiki/Organism>.

5. "Terms. Organism." About Got it. Accessed 11 March 2007. <http://www.cs.uu.nl/people/ronnie/local/genome/o.html>.

6. "Embryo." Online Etymology Dictionary. Douglas Harper, Historian. Accessed 13 Mar. 2007. <http://dictionary.reference.com/browse/embryo>.

7. "Embryo." Dictionary.com Unabridged (v 1.1). Random House, Inc. Accessed 13 Mar. 2007. <Dictionary.com http://dictionary.reference.com/browse/embryo>.

8. "Embryo." Merriam Webster Online. Accessed 13 March 2007. <http://209.161.33.50/dictionary/embryo>.

9. "Embryo." The American Heritage® Dictionary of the English Language, Fourth Edition. Houghton Mifflin Company, 2004. Accessed 13 Mar. 2007. Dictionary.com <http://dictionary.reference.com/browse/embryo>.

10. "Embryo." Glossary of Stem Cell Science Terms. Harvard Stem Cell Institute. Accessed 13 March 2007. <http://www.hsci.harvard.edu/glossary>.

11. Bush, George. "Fact Sheet." United States Department of Human Health and Services. 14 July 2004. Accessed 9 August 2006. <http://www.hhs.gov/news/press/2004pres/20040714b.html>.

12. "Israel Leads the Way on Stem Cells." The Jewish Daily Forward. 25 August 2006. Accessed March 2007. <http://www.forward.com/articles/israel-leads-the-way-on-stem-cells/>.

13. Kessler, John A. "Stem Cells I want to see my daughter walk again." Accessed 27 December 2006.

Chapter Three

14. "Cooperators of Opus Dei." The Catholic Resource Network. Accessed 5 February 2007. <http://www.ewtn.com/library/SPIRIT/ODCOOP.TXT>.

15. Alterman, Eric. "Neoconning the Media A Very Short History of Neoconservatism." Media Transparency. April 22, 2005. Accessed 4 February 2007. <http://www.mediatransparency.org/story.php?storyID=2>.

16. Frank Cocozzelli. "Neoconservatism, the Catholic Church And Stem Cells Attack on Science." Talk2action.org. Accessed 15 October 2006. <http://www.talk2action.org/story/2006/10/15/151651/45>.

Chapter Four

17. "United States is not a Christian Nation." Embassy of Heaven. Accessed 6 March 2007. <http://secular. embassyofheaven.com/usa/tripoli.htm>.

18. "Treaty of Tripoli." Wikipedia. Accessed 6 March 2007. <http://en.wikipedia.org/wiki/Treaty_of_Tripoli>.

Chapter Five

19. "Text of President Bush's announcement Thursday in Crawford, Texas." Accessed 4 December 2006. <http:// www.nrlc.org/Killing_Embryos/textpresidentbush.htm>.

20. Faden, Ruth R. and John D. Gearhart. "Facts on Stem Cells." Washington Post. 23 August 2004. Accessed 10 January 2007. <http://www.washingtonpost.com/wp-dyn/articles/A25071-2004Aug22.html>.

21. "Stem cell debate goes to voters." Stateline.org. 5 October 2006. Accessed 30 November 2006. <http://www.stateline. org/live/details/story?contentId=146780>.

22. Cocozzelli, Frank. "Pro-Life, Pro-Tobacco—Anti-Stem Cell Research?" Email # 310 from Don C. Reed. 26 March 2007.

23. Easton, Susan. "Annotated Bibliography of Resources on Spirituality and Health." Accessed 6 April 2007. <http:// s89864416.onlinehome.us/seaston/healthbib.htm>.

24. "Text of President Bush's Announcement Thursday in Crawford, Texas." 4 December 2006. <http://www.nrlc. org/Killing_Embryos/textpresidentbush.htm>.

25. Faden, Ruth R. and John D. Gearhart. "Facts on Stem Cells." The Washington Post. 23 August 2004. Accessed

10 January 2007. <http://www.washingtonpost.com/wp-dyn/articles/A25071-2004Aug22.html>.

26. Bailey, Ronald. "More Stubborn Facts Are embryos people?" National Review. 6 August 2001. Accessed 9 August 2006. <http://www.nationalreview.com/comment/comment-bailey080601.shtml>.

Chapter Six

27. Bush, George W. "President Bush on Cloning." PBS.org. 10 April 2002. Accessed 9 August 2006. <http://www.pbs.org/newshour/updates/april02/bush-cloning_4-10.html>.

28. Reed, Don C. Email to Listserv. 21 February 2007.

29. Carter, Jimmy. "Stem Cell News." CAMR. 22 February 2007. <http://www.camradvocacy.org/news_detail.aspx?id=SArch13>.

30. Ford, Gerald. "Stem Cell News." CAMR. 25 April 2002. <http://www.camradvocacy.org/news_detail.aspx?id=SArch14>.

Chapter Seven

31. Reed, Don C. "McNerney in the Morning." Stem Cell Battles. 24 October 2006. <http://www.stemcellbattles.com/Archive%20242_10-24-06%20-%20MCNERNEY%20IN%20THE%20MORNING.htm>.

32. Dwyer, Sheila. "Dr. Evan Snyder Discusses Advances in A-T Research." August 18, 2000. Accessed 11 December 2006. <http://www.body1.com/hero/index.cfm/1/16/1>.

33. Saltus, Richard. "The Man Who Fixes Brains / Conference Calendar Deadline Friday." The Boston Globe. 27

December 2006. <http://www.pdcaregiver.org/StemCell.html>.

34. "Boy's Mom Fights for His 'RIGHT TO RECOVER', Stem-Cell Debate's Fate Could Fall to Voters." 5 March 2007. Accessed 8 March 2007. Orlando Sentinel. <http://www.orlandosentinel.com/news/orl-mstemcells0507mar05,0,7110019.story?page=2&coll=orl-news-headlines>.

35. **"Gov. Blagojevich announces recipients of $5 million in new state Stem Cell Research funding." Illinois Regenerative Medicine Institute. 17 August 2006. Accessed 3 April 2007. <http://www.idph.state.il.us/irmi/news_081706.html>.**

36. "Statement of Support for Stem Cell Research." 17 July 2006. Accessed 3 January 2007. <http://obama.senate.gov/speech/060717-statement_of_support_for_stem_cell_research/index.html>.

37. "Governor Doyle Announces $1 Million for Stem Cell Start-up Company." Office of the Governor Jim Doyle. 10 October 2006. Accessed 28 December 2006. <http://www.wisgov.state.wi.us/journal_media_detail.asp?locid=19&prid=2362>.

Chapter Eight

38. "Israel Leads the Way on Stem Cells." The Jewish Daily Forward. 25 August 2006. Accessed March 2007. <http://www.forward.com/articles/israel-leads-the-way-on-stem-cells/>.

39. Kraft, Dina. "Stem Cell Researchers in Israel warily eye debate in Washington." Deep South Jewish Voice. 16 June 2005. Accessed 4 December 2006. <http://deepsouthjewishvoice.blogspot.com/2005/06/israel-file-stem-cell-researchers-in.html>.

40. Einhorn, Bruce and Jennifer Veale and Manjeet Kripalani. "Asia Is Stem Cell Central, Singapore and others are racing to grab the lead in a promising field." Business Week Online. 10 January 2005. 27 December 2006. <http://www.businessweek.com/magazine/content/05_02/b3915052.htm>.

Chapter Nine

41. Campo-Flores, Arian. "Split Remains." Newsweek. Aug 26, 2006. MSNBC.com. Accessed 7 November 2006. <http://www.msnbc.msn.com/id/14527419/site/newsweek/>.

42. Campo-Flores, Arian. "Those Favoring Stem Cell Research Increases to a 73 to 11 Percent Majority." Washington Post-ABC News Poll. The Washington Post, Jan.20, 3006. Assessed 21 January 2007.<http://www.washingtonpost.com/wp-srv/politics/polls/postpoll_012007.htm>.

43. Doerflinger, Richard M. "Science and Ethics: Together Again?" United States Conference of Catholic Bishops. 26 August 2005 Accessed 3 April 2007. <http://www.usccb.org/prolife/publicat/lifeissues/082605.shtml>.

44. Stolberg, Sheryl Gay. "Senate's Leader Veers From Bush Over Stem Cells." The New York Times. 29 July 2005. Accessed 30 November 2006. <http://www.nytimes.com/2005/07/29/politics/29stem.html?ex=1280289600&en=b97f268f2f13d8d9&ei=5088&partner=rssnyt&emc=rss>.

45. Reagan, Mike and Howard Dean, M.D. "Stem Cell Pro and Con." MSNBC.com. 12 December 2006. <http://cagle.msnbc.com/news/StemCellsProCon/main.asp>.

46. "Pelosi: A Bush Veto of Stem Cell Legislation Will Say 'No' to Hope for Millions of American Families." Congresswoman Nancy Pelosi. July 19, 2006. Accessed 29

November, 2006. <http://www.house.gov/pelosi/press/releases/July06/StemCellVeto.html>.

47. "U.S. Senate Roll Call Votes 109th Congress - 2nd Session." United States Senate. 10 October 2006. <http://www.senate.gov/legislative/LIS/roll_call_lists/roll_call_vote_cfm.cfm?congress=109&session=2&vote=00206>.

Chapter Ten

48. "Stem Cell Research Enhancement Act of 2005 (Enrolled as Agreed to or Passed by Both House and Senate) H.R.810." The Library of Congress. <http://thomas.loc.gov/cgi-bin/query/D?c109:5:./temp/~c109JhWf1X::>.

49. "US Governs by 'Coercion,' Iran Leader Writes in Open Letter to Americans, Ahmadinejad Urges Pullout from Iraq." MSNBC News Services. Nov 29, 2006. <http://www.msnbc.msn.com/id/15947213/>.

50. Bush, George W. "President Discusses Stem Cell Research." The White House. 9 August 2001. Accessed 1 December 2006. <http://www.whitehouse.gov/news/releases/2001/08/20010809-2.html>.

51. Reed, Don C. "Shocking Conversation." Email to listserv. 21 March 2007.

52. "Researcher: Keep Embryonic Stem Cell Work Anthony Atala Tells Congress His Amniotic Fluid Work no Reason to Stop Embryonic Research." CBS News. 9 January 2007. Accessed 22 February 2007. <http://www.cbsnews.com/stories/2007/01/09/health/main2339877.shtml>.

53. "In Case You Want the Unbiased, Bipartisan Truth: Embryonic Stem Cell Research Shows Great Promise." Texans for Advancement of Medical Research. 22 February 2007. <http://www.txamr.org/index.php?option=com_content&task=view&id=212&Itemid=1>.

54. Kessler, John A. "Stem Cells I want to see my daughter walk again." Chicago Tribune. June 2004. Accessed 27 December 2006.

Chapter Eleven

55. Republican Study Committee. "H.R. 3 — Stem Cell Research Enhancement Act of 2007." Legislative Bulletin. January 11, 2007. 20 February 2007. <http://www.house.gov/hensarling/rsc/lgbullettins07.shtml>.

56. Smith, Shane Dr., William Neaves and Steven Teitelbaum. "Adult Stem Cell Treatments for Disease?" Science Magazine Vol. 313, p.439, 28 July 2006. 4 February 2007.

57. Kleinfeld, Sarah, David Prentice and Bill Saunders. "Adult Stem Cell Success Stories – 2006." Family Research Council. 20 February 2007. <http://www.frc.org/get.cfm?i=IS06H01>.

58. "Stem Cells, The White House And Rankled Researchers." The Washington Post. 22 January 2007. 22 February 2007. <http://www.washingtonpost.com/wp-dyn/content/article/2007/01/21/AR2007012100761.html>.

59. Goldstein, Lawrence S.B. Paul Berg and George Q. Daley. "Stem Cell 'Alternatives' Fog the Debate." 19 July 2005, Page A21. The Washington Post. <http://www.washingtonpost.com/wp-dyn/content/article/2005/07/18/AR2005071801323.html?referrer=emailarticle>.

60. Reed, Don C. email to listserv # 297 Wednesday, 21 February 2007 "Iowa Stem Cell Emergency."

61. Smith, Shane G. "Research with Adult and Embryonic Cells is Essential." 9 January 2007. Accessed 4 February 2007. Op. Ed in St. Louis Dispatch. PDF from author.

62. "Letter to Members of Congress." January 9, 2007. <http://harkin.senate.gov/documents/pdf/StemCell110th.pdf>.

Chapter Twelve

63. Kessler, John A. "Stem Cells I want to see my daughter walk again." Chicago Tribune. June 2004. Accessed 27 December 2006.

64. Conner, Steve. "Hawking Criticizes EU States Trying to Ban Stem Cell Research." The Independent Online. 24 July 2006. <http://news.independent.co.uk/world/science_technology/article1193119.ece>.

65. "The Potential for Stem Cell Cures and Therapies." California Stem Cell Research and Cures Initiative YES on 71: Coalition for Stem Cell Research and Cures, #1260661. PDF from Shane G. Smith. 3 April 2007.

66. Somers, Terri. "How Prop. 71 Came to Life, California Stem Cell Research and Cures Act was Work of Eclectic Group that Included Film Director, Finance Expert, Republican and Researcher." The San Diego Union-Tribune. 19 December 2004. Accessed 3 April 2007. <http://www.signonsandiego.com/uniontrib/20041219/news_1n19stemcell.html>.

67. Reagan, Mike and Howard Dean, M.D. "Stem Cell Pro and Con." MSNBC.com. 12 December 2006. <http://cagle.msnbc.com/news/StemCellsProCon/main.asp>.

68. Zuckman, Jill. "Will Stem Cells be the Key in Races?" Chicago Tribune. 24 October 2006. Accessed 1 March 2007. <http://deseretnews.com/dn/view/0,1249,650201249,00.html>.

69. Dwyer, Sheila. "Dr. Evan Snyder Discusses Advances in A-T Research." Body1.com. August 18, 2000. Accessed 11 December 2006. <http://www.body1.com/hero/index.

cfm/1/16/1>.

70. Kessler, John A. "Stem Cells I want to see my daughter walk again." <u>Chicago Tribune</u>. June 2004. Accessed 27 December 2006.

Chapter Thirteen

71. Saltus, Richard. "The Man Who Fixes Brains / Conference Calendar Deadline Friday." <u>The Boston Globe.</u> 27 December 2006. <http://www.pdcaregiver.org/StemCell.html>.

BIBLIOGRAPHY A

"$181 Million Headed for Stem Cell Institute." California Institute for Regenerative Medicine. 20 November 2006. 28 December 2006. <http://www.cirm.ca.gov/pressreleases/2006/11/11-20-06.asp>.

"A new start." Arthritis Research Campaign. 9 January 2007. <http://www.arc.org.uk/newsviews/arctdy/111/stemcells.htm>.

"About us." Aldagen. 3 January 2007. <http://www.aldagen.com/a_about.htm>.

"Advances in Sweden's Human Embryonic Stem Cell Research." Cell News. 26 August 2004. 26 December 2006. <http://www.geocities.com/giantfideli/art/CellNEWS_Adv_Swed_hESC.html>.

"Advising the President on Ethical Issues Related to Advances in Biomedical Science and Technology." The President's Council on Bioethics. 10 September 2006. <www.bioethics.gov>.

"Albert Einstein: God, Religion & Theology." Space and Motion. 13 March 2007. <http://www.spaceandmotion.com/albert-einstein-god-religion-theology.htm>.

"America not Founded on Christian Principles; Bible Rejected as Word of God by Founders." Arizona State University State Press, April 29, 1986, vol. 68, no. 132. 26 November 2006. <http://www.discord.org/~lippard/state-press-19860429.html>.

"Americans with Disabilities: 2002 - Table A." U.S. Census Bureau. 30 November 2006. <http://www.census.gov/hhes/www/disability/sipp/disab02/ds02ta.html>.

"Amniotic Fluid of Pregnant Women as an Alternative Stem Cell Source." Stem Cell Research. 9 January 2007. <http://www.stemnews.com/archives/001437.html>.

"Approval Granted for Harvard Stem Cell Institute Researchers to Attempt Creation of Disease-Specific Embryonic Stem Cell Lines." Harvard University Gazette. 6 June 2006. 25 March 2006. <http://www.news.harvard.edu/gazette/daily/2006/06/06-stemcell.html>.

"Benjamin Franklin." The War on Faith. 26 November 2006. <http://thewaronfaith.com/ff_franklin.htm>.

"Bone Marrow Holds Promise in Treatment of MS." The Multiple Sclerosis Resource Centre 9 January 2007. <http://www.msrc.co.uk/index.cfm?fuseaction=show&pageid=1331>.

"Bone Marrow Stem Cells Help Mend Broken Hearts." BioEd Online. 3 January 2007. <http://www.bioedonline.org/news/news.cfm?art=936>.

"Boy's Mom Fights for His 'Right To Recover', Stem-Cell Debate's Fate Could Fall to Voters." 8 March 2007. Orlando Sentinel. <http://www.orlandosentinel.com/news/orl-mstemcells0507mar05,0,7110019.story?page=2&coll=orl-news-headlines>.

"BresaGen's Success Promises Much to Many." AusIndustry. 2 January 2007. <http://www.ausindustry.gov.au/content/content.cfm?ObjectID=DB3BF7E5-498F-458E-A3BCD47DDD575922&L3Keyword=stem%20cell>.

"California Stem Cell Board Approves Terms for Grants to For-Profit Research Entities." California Institute for Regenerative Medicine. 7 December 2006. 28 December 2006. <http://www.cirm.ca.gov/pressreleases/2006/12/12-07-06.asp>.

"California Stem Cell Board to Consider Requirements for Grants to For-Profit Research Entities." California Institute for Regenerative Medicine. 5 December 2006. 28 December 2006. <http://www.cirm.ca.gov/pressreleases/2006/12/12-05-06.asp>.

"Causes of MS." Multiple Sclerosis International Federation." 9 January 2007. <http://www.msif.org/en/ms_the_disease/causes_of_ms.html>.

"Children's Neurobiological Solutions Foundation CNS Foundation Joins A-TCP in Funding Stem Cell Based Therapies." CNS Foundation. 8 January 2007. <http://www.cnsfoundation.org>.

"Christianity." Religious Tolerance.org 18 December 2006. <http://www.religioustolerance.org/christ.htm>.

"Chronic Granulomatous Disease." 9 January 2007. Wikipedia. <http://en.wikipedia.org/wiki/Chronic_granulomatous_disease>.

"Clinically Significant Results Seen in Cerebral Palsy in Children." Steenblock Research Institute. 9 January 2007. <http://www.14ushop.com/wizard/push-is-on-revised8704.html>.

"Cloning's Out, but Stem Cell R&D Will Have Rules." The Times of India. 27 December 2006. <http://timesofindia.indiatimes.com/NEWS/India/Clonings_out_but_stem_cell_RD_will_have_rules/articleshow/461473.cms>.

"Colorado's Advance on Stem Cell Research." DenverPost.com. 24 August 2006. 28 December 2006. <http://www.denverpost.com/editorials/ci_4233782>.

"Company Profile." ES Cell International. 28 December 2006. <http://www.escellinternational.com/aboutus/companyprofile.htm>.

"Company." Neuronova.com. 1 January 2007. <http://www.neuronova.com/section.php?node=%3C0%3E>.

"Cooperators of Opus Dei." The Catholic Resource Network. 5 February 2007. <http://www.ewtn.com/library/SPIRIT/ODCOOP.TXT>.

"Court Upholds Constitutionality of Stem Cell Program, Judge Sabraw Declares Proposition 71 Constitutional in its Entirety." California Institutes for Regenerative Medicine. 21 April 2006. 11 December 2006. <http://www.cirm.ca.gov/pressreleases/2006/04/04-21-06.asp>.

"December 18, 2006 Commission Unveils Guidelines, Applications for New Stem Cell Research Grant Program." State of New Jersey Commission on Science and Technology. 18 December 2006. 29 December 2006. <http://www.state.nj.us/scitech/about/news/approved/20061218.html>.

"Definition of Organism." Yahoo Education. 11 March 2007. <http://education.yahoo.com/reference/dictionary/entry/organism>.

"Difference Between Private and Public Cord Blood Banking." Stem Cell Research. 9 January 2007. <http://www.stemnews.com/archives/001434.html>.

"Disgraced Stem Cell Scientist Indicted for Fraud." The Turkish Weekly. 6 December 2006. <http://www.turkishweekly.net/news.php?id=31698>.

"Dr. Hwang and the Bad Apple Theory of Scientific Misconduct." 25 December 2005. 6 December 2006. <http://blog.bioethics.net/2005/12/dr-hwang-and-bad-apple-theory-of.html>.

"Early Stages of the Establishment of Christianity." Religious Book for Seekers. 23 October 2006. <http://www.religiousbook.net/Books/Online_books/Sh/Heart_20.html>.

"EFF Analysis of the Provisions of the USA Patriot Act." Electronic Frontier Foundation. 27 October 2003. 29 November, 2006. <http://www.eff.org/Privacy/Surveillance/Terrorism/20011031_eff_usa_patriot_analysis.php>.

"Elizabeth Blackburn, Fired by President Bush from Bioethics Commission, Awarded Franklin Medal." 20 March 2005. Accessed 27 March 2007. Bioethics.net. < http://blog.bioethics.net/2005/03/elizabeth-blackburn-fired-by-president.html l>.

"Embryo." Dictionary.com Unabridged (v 1.1). Random House, Inc. Accessed 13 Mar. 2007. <http://dictionary.reference.com/ browse/embryo>.

"Embryo." Glossary of Stem Cell Science Terms. Harvard Stem Cell Institute. Accessed13 March 2007. <http://www.hsci.harvard. edu/glossary>.

"Embryo." Merriam Webster Online. Accessed 13 March 2007. <http://209.161.33.50/dictionary/embryo>.

"Embryo." Online Etymology Dictionary. Douglas Harper, Historian. Accessed 13 Mar. 2007. <http://dictionary.reference.com/ browse/embryo>.

"Embryo." The American Heritage® Dictionary of the English Language, Fourth Edition. Houghton Mifflin Company, 2004. Accessed 13 March 2007._<http://dictionary.reference.com/ browse/embryo>.

"Embryonic Stem Cells." BioEd Online Baylor College of Medicine. 9 January 2007. <http://www.bioedonline.org/slides/tray_act. cfm?q=embryonic+stem+cells&dpg=4&act=dl >.

"Episode 6: Miracle Cell." PBS. 15 December 2006. <http://www.pbs. org/wnet/innovation/about_episode6.html>.

"Global Positions in Stem Cell Research." UK Stem Cell Initiative. 24 November 2005. 6 December 2006. <http://www. advisorybodies.doh.gov.uk/uksci/global/czechrepublic.htm>.

"Glossary of Selected Terms." Science and Technology/Engineering._ Curriculum Framework. 11 March 2007. <http://www.doe. mass.edu/frameworks/scitech/2001/resources/glossary. html>.

"Glossary of Stem Cell Science Terms." Harvard Stem Cell Institute. 25 November 2007. <http://stemcell.harvard.edu/glossary>.

"Governor Doyle Announces $1 Million for Stem Cell Start-up Company." Office of the Governor Jim Doyle. 10 October 2006. Accessed 28 December 2006. <http://www.wisgov.state.wi.us/journal_media_detail.asp?locid=19&prid=2362>.

"Governor Schwarzenegger Nominates Chair and Vice Chair of Stem Cell Oversight Committee and Appoints Five Committee Members." Schwarzenegger.com. 13 December 2004. <http://www.schwarzenegger.com/news.asp?id=1832>.

"H.R.810—The Stem Cell Research Enhancement Act of 2005." Office of Legislative Policy and Analysis. 20 August, 2006. <http://olpa.od.nih.gov/tracking/109/house_bills/session1/hr-810.asp>.

"Harvard's Dr. Evan Snyder to Head the "Manhattan Project" of stem-cell research." Cure ALS Ride for life online. 22 November 2003. 5 September 2006. <http://www.rideforlife.com/archives/000728.html>.

"Human Embryonic Stem Cell Research in China." U.S. Embassy. 27 December 2006. <http://www.usembassy-china.org.cn/sandt/stemcell.htm>.

"Hwang Woo-Suk." Wikipedia. Answers.com. 6 December 2006. <http://www.answers.com/topic/hwang-woo-suk>.

"Ill. Senate OKs Stem Cell Research." 23 February 2007. Associated Press. <http://hosted.ap.org/dynamic/stories/I/ILLINOIS_STEM_CELLS?SITE=FLROC&SECTION=US&TEMPLATE=DEFAULT.>.

"In Case You Want the Unbiased, Bipartisan Truth: Embryonic Stem Cell Research Shows Great Promise." Texans for Advancement of Medical Research. 22 February 2007. <http://www.txamr.org/index.php?option=com_content&task=view&id=212&Itemid=1>.

"Indian Stem Cell Research Would be Guided by an Appropriate Strategy in Near Future." 11 December 2006. Taragana. <http://stemcell.taragana.net/archive/indian-stem-cell-research-shall-be-guided-by-an-appropriate-strategy/>.

"International Legislation on Human Embryonic Stem Cell Research." International Society for Stem Cell Research. 4 January 2007. <http://isscr.org/public/regions/index.cfm>.

"International Policies on Stem Cell Research." MBBnet. 27 December 2006. <http://mbbnet.umn.edu/scmap.html>.

"Introduction: Ataxia Telangiectasia." Wrong Diagnosis. 5 January 2007. <http://www.wrongdiagnosis.com/a/ataxia_telangiectasia/intro.htm>.

"Israel Leads the Way on Stem Cells." The Jewish Daily Forward. 25 August 2006. Accessed March 2007. <http://www.forward.com/articles/israel-leads-the-way-on-stem-cells/>.

"Issues and Procedures in Women's Health Molar Pregnancy." OBGYN.net. 25 January 2007. <http://www.obgyn.net/women/women.asp?page=/women/articles/molarpreg_dah>.

"JDRF Issues New Stem Cell Research Q&A." Juvenile Diabetes Research Foundation.. 22 March 2000. 13 December 2006. <http://www.jdrf.org/index.cfm?page_id=102094>.

"John Adams." America's Founding Fathers and Christianity. 26 November 2006. <http://afgen.com/church2a.html>.

"Learn More about Stem Cells." Wisconsin Stem Cell Now Inc. 2 January 2007. <http://www.wistemcellnow.org/pages/learn.html>.

"Letter to Members of Congress." January 9, 2007. <http://harkin.senate.gov/documents/pdf/StemCell110th.pdf>.

"Mesoblast." Mesoblast Adult Stem Cell Company. 19 December 2006. <http://www.mesoblast.com/>.

"Monitoring Stem Cell Research: Current Federal Law and Policy." The President's Council on Bioethics.10 September 2006. <http://bioethics.gov/reports/stemcell/chapter1.html>.

"Monitoring Stem Cell Research: Notes on Early Human Development." The President's Council on Bioethics. 10 September 2006. <http://bioethics.gov/reports/stemcell/appendix_a.html>.

"Mutant Mice Show Key Autism Traits." Science Daily. 9 January 2007. <http://www.sciencedaily.com/releases/2006/05/060503203122.htm>.

"Nancy Reagan Endorses Human Embryonic Research." Medical News Today. 10 May 2004 12 December 2006. <http://www.medicalnewstoday.com/medicalnews.php?newsid=8128>.

"Nancy Reagan Plea on Stem Cells." BBC News. 10 May, 2004. 12 December 2006. <http://news.bbc.co.uk/2/hi/americas/3700015.stm>.

"National Institutes of Health and ES Cell International Pte. Ltd Sign International Stem Cell Research Agreement." 11 April 2002. NIH News Release. 28 December 2006. <http://www.nih.gov/news/pr/apr2002/od-11.htm>.

"New Paper Challenges Statistical Design and Conclusions of Amgen's Phase II GDNF Study." GRC Issue: GDNF Research. 4 August 2006. Accessed 20 February 2007. <http://www.grassrootsconnection.com/grcissue_GDNF_research.htm>.

"NIH Grants Infrastructure Award for Embryonic Stem Cell Research to ES Cell International." National Institutes of Health. April 26, 2002. 22 January 2007. <http://www.nih.gov/news/pr/apr2002/od-26d.htm>.

"NIH Guidelines." AAAS Center for Science, Technology, and Congress. 26 December 2006. <http://www.aaas.org/spp/cstc/briefs/stemcells/index.shtml#guidelines>.

"Novel Stem Cell Technology Develops a New Cell for Repairing Spinal Cord Injuries." The Quad Link. 28 April 2006. 24 October 2006. <.http://thequadlink.iwonpages.com/page/txzt/Banner_Ads.html>.

"Novel Stem Cell Technology Leads to Better Spinal Cord Repair."
Medilexicon. 24 October 2006. <http://www.medilexicon.
com/medicalnews.php?newsid=42430>.

"Older Stem Cells Don't Just Wear Out, They Actively Shut
Themselves Down." University of Michigan. <http://www.
umich.edu/news/index.html?Releases/2006/Sep06/r090606>.

"Organism." Wikipedia. 11 March 2007. <http://en.wikipedia.org/
wiki/Organism>.

"Osteoporosis." Alliance for Stem Cell Research. 8 January 2007.
<http://www.curesforcalifornia.com/page.php?id=111>.

"Our Christian Nation." Biosfear. 24 August 2005. 26 November 2006.
<http://www.biosfear.com/archives/000165.html>.

"Overview of GDNF." Parkinson's Pipeline Project. 20 February 2007.
<http://www.pdpipeline.org/advocacy/gdnf_overview.htm>.

"Part of the Immune System is Missing." NIAID and NIH. 8 January
2007. <http://www.niaid.nih.gov/final/immds/immdef.htm>.

"Partial Molar Pregnancy." Health Information Center at the Cleveland
Clinic. 25 January 2007. <http://www.clevelandclinic.org/
health/health-info/docs/3800/3867.asp?index=12332&src=n
ewsp>.

"Pelosi: A Bush Veto of Stem Cell Legislation Will Say 'No' to Hope
for Millions of American Families." Congresswoman Nancy
Pelosi. July 19, 2006. Accessed 29 November, 2006. <http://
www.house.gov/pelosi/press/releases/July06/StemCellVeto.
html>.

"Pentagon Sees U.S. War Cost in Iraq Rising." 19 January 2007. Reuters.
<http://in.today.reuters.com/news/newsArticle.aspx?type=
worldNews&storyID=2007-01-19T072608Z_01_NOOTR_
RTRJONC_0_India-284211-1.xml&archived=False>.

"Plaintiffs Robert Suthers and Niwana Martin's Memorandum of Law in Support of their Motion for a Preliminary Injunction." gdnf4parkinsons.org. 25 April 2005. Accessed 3 March 2007. <http://www.gdnf4parkinsons.org/LEGALMEMO.html>.

"Poll: Stem Cell Use Gains Support." CBS News Polls. May 24, 2005. 25 October 2006. http://www.cbsnews.com/ stories/2005/05/24/opinion/polls/main697546.shtml.

"Polls Show Strong Support for Stem Cell Research." CAMR. 4 December 2006. <http://www.jdrf.org/files/Advocacy/Stem_ Cell_Info/ESCPollInfo.pdf>.

"Protestantism." Wikipedia. 18 December 2006. <http://en.wikipedia. org/wiki/Protestant>.

"Public Backs Stem Cell Research Most Say Government Should Fund Use of Embryos." ABCNews online. 27 November 2006. <http://www.abcnews.go.com/sections/politics/DailyNews/ poll010626.html>.

"Reformation." About.com. 18 December 2006. <http://atheism. about.com/library/glossary/western/bldef_reformation.htm>.

"Research on Umbilical Cord Stem Cells and Autism." Stem Cell Therapies. 8 January 2007. <http://www.stemcelltherapies. org/umresearch/autism-research.html>.

"Researcher: Keep Embryonic Stem Cell Work Anthony Atala Tells Congress His Amniotic Fluid Work No Reason To Stop Embryonic Research." CBS News. 9 January 2007. 22 February 2007. <http://www.cbsnews.com/stories/2007/01/09/ health/main2339877.shtml>.

"Researchers Turn Cord Blood into Lung Cells." Science Daily. November 13, 2006. 13 December 2006. http://www. sciencedaily.com/releases/2006/11/061101150949.htm

"Ron Reagan to Address Democratic Convention." MSNBC.com. 12 July 2004. 29 November 2006. <http://www.msnbc.msn.com/ id/5425570/>.

"Scientists Describe How Chemical Turns Progenitor Stem Cells into Bone Cells." Medical News Toady. 6 September 2004. 8 January 2007. <http://www.medicalnewstoday.com/medicalnews.php?newsid=12975>.

"Select Global Stem Cell Research Centers." University of Minnesota Medical School MBBNet. 6 December 2006. <http://www.mbbnet.umn.edu/scmap/scresearchmap.html>.

"Senator Feinstein Urges Senate Leaders to Take up Stem Cell Bill." U.S. Senator Dianne Feinstein. May 25, 2005. 30 November 2006. <http://feinstein.senate.gov/05releases/r-stemcll-nuser525.htm>.

"Septugint." Septugint. 18 December 2006. <http://www.septuagint.net/>.

"Someday, Maybe, Repairs for Spines and Brains." CNN.com Health. 6 November 2000. 20 August, 2006. <http://archives.cnn.com/2000/HEALTH/11/06/fixing.spines.ap/index.html>.

"South Africa Set to Have Africa's First Stem Cell Bank." Stem Cell Network. 3 January 2006. <http://www.stemcellnetwork.ca/news/articles.php?id=586>.

"Spinal Cord Injury Facts and Figures at a Glance June 2006." Spinal Cord Injury Information Network. 20 August, 2006. <http://www.spinalcord.uab.edu/show.asp?durki=21446>.

"Statement of Support for Stem Cell Research." 17 July 2006. 3 January 2007. Senator Obama. <http://obama.senate.gov/speech/060717-statement_of_support_for_stem_cell_research/index.html>.

"Stem Cell Bone Repair Trials Produce Outstanding Results." Mesoblast Adult Stem Cell Company. 6 September, 2006. <http://www.google.com/search?hl=en&q=Mesoblast%27s+First+Stem+Cell+Patient+Walks+Unaided&btnG=Google+Search>.

"Stem Cell Debate Goes to Voters." Stateline.org. 5 October 2006. 30
        November 2006. <http://www.stateline.org/live/details/story
        ?contentId=146780>.

"Stem Cell Research Action by State." Stem Cell Action Network. 2
        January 2007. <http://www.stemcellpage.com/index_files/
        stemcellactionbystate.htm>.

"Stem Cell Research Enhancement Act of 2005 (Enrolled as Agreed to
        or Passed by Both House and Senate) H.R.810." The Library
        of Congress. <http://thomas.loc.gov>.

"Stem Cell Research." Science and Nature (FOX). Accessed 20 March
        2007. <http://www.pollingreport.com/science.htm>.

"Stem Cell Research." The Pew Forum on Religion & Public
        Life. 4 December 2006. <http://pewforum.org/docs/
        ?DocID=149>.

"Stem Cell Support in Patients with Rheumatoid Arthritis."
        ClinicalTrials.gov. 9 January 2007. <http://www.clinicaltrials.
        gov/ct/show/NCT00278551 >.

"Stem Cell Therapy Helps MS Woman." BBC News. 9 January 2007.
        <http://news.bbc.co.uk/1/hi/scotland/4442836.stm>.

"Stem Cell Therapy in Multiple Sclerosis - Now it is Time to Really
        Start." Multiple Sclerosis Resource Center. 9 January 2007.
        <http://www.msrc.co.uk/index.cfm?fuseaction=show&pageid
        =1405>.

"Stem Cells an Unlikely Therapy for Alzheimer's" The Washington
        Post Company. 10 June 2004. 12 December 2006. <http://
        www.washingtonpost.com/wp-dyn/articles/A29561-2004Jun9.
        html>.

"Stem Cells and Diabetes." The National Institutes of Health. 13
        December 2006. <http://stemcells.nih.gov/info/scireport/
        chapter7.asp>.

"Stem Cells and Government Archives." Stem Cell Research Medical Health News. 30 <November 2006. http://www.stemnews. com/archives/stem cells-and-government.html>.

"Stem Cells to be Tested in Repairing Heart Muscle." Cord blood Registry. 3 January 2007. <http://www.cordblood.com/cord_ blood_news/stem_cell_news/a_stem_heart_test.asp>.

"Stem Cells, Inc. Geron Shares Surge on Promising Stem Cell Findings." Stem Cell Business News. 2 May 2003. Accessed 9 January 2007. <http://www.ferghanapartners. com/articles/StemCellBusinessNewsMay22003/ StemCellSectorNeedsaViableProducttoSparkInvestorInterest. pdf#search='Stem%20Cell%20for%20quad%20recovery>.

"Stem Cells, The White House and Rankled Researchers." The Washington Post. 22 January 2007. Accessed 22 February 2007. <http://www.washingtonpost.com/wp-dyn/content/ article/2007/01/21/AR2007012100761.html>.

"Stem-Cell Debate Turns Deadly Dumb." Denver Post online. 29 December 2006. <http://blogs.denverpost.com/ washington/2006/07/21/stem-cell-debate-turns-deadly- dumb/>.

"Stem-Cell Transplants: A Cure for Arthritis?" Arthritis Foundation. 8 January 2007. <http://www.arthritis.org/resources/news/ news_stemupdate.asp>.

"Symptoms." Arthritis Foundation. 9 January 2007. <http://www. arthritis.org/conditions/DiseaseCenter/RA/ra_symptoms. asp>.

"Tell Congress: Vote for Stem Cell Research." StemPAC. 11 January 2007. <http://www.stempac.com/>.

"Terms. Organism." About Got it. 11 March 2007. <http://www.cs.uu. nl/people/ronnie/local/genome/o.html>.

"Text of President Bush's Announcement Thursday in Crawford, Texas." 4 December 2006. <http://www.nrlc.org/Killing_ Embryos/textpresidentbush.htm>.

"Text of Proposed Laws, Proposition 71." 11 December 2006. CIRM. <http://www.cirm.ca.gov/prop71/pdf/prop71.pdf>.

"The History of the Septuagint, and its Terminology." 18 December 2006. <http://www.kalvesmaki.com/LXX/>.

"The Modern Faces of the Horned God." 4 December 2006. <http://www.lugodoc.demon.co.uk/newgods.htm>.

"The Nicene Creed." 24 October, 2006. <http://www.iclnet.org/pub/resources/text/history/creed.nicene.txt>.

"Therapeutic Approach." Stem Cell Therapeutics. 23 January 2007. <http://www.stemcellthera.com/>.

"Thomas Jefferson & Christianity." America's Founding Fathers and Christianity. 26 November 2006. <http://afgen.com/church2a.html>.

"Totipotency." 21 December 2006. Wikipedia. <http://en.wikipedia.org/wiki/Totipotency>.

"Transplantation of Human Embryonic Stem Cell-Derived Cells to a Rat Model of Parkinson's Disease: Effect of In Vitro Differentiation on Graft Survival and Teratoma Formation." Stem Cells International Journal. 26 December 2006. <http://stemcells.alphamedpress.org/cgi/content/abstract/24/6/1433>.

"Treaty of Tripoli." Wikipedia. 6 March 2007. <http://en.wikipedia.org/wiki/Treaty_of_Tripoli>.

"U.S. Senate Roll Call Votes 109th Congress - 2nd Session." United States Senate. 10 October 2006. <http://www.senate.gov/legislative/LIS/roll_call_lists/roll_call_vote_cfm.cfm?congress=109&session=2&vote=00206>.

"U.S. Stem Cell Patent Issued." Phosita: An Intellectual Property Law Blog. Posted 23 August 2004. Accessed 27 March 2007. <http://www.okpatents.com/phosita/archives/ip_public_policy/>.

"UCSF Faculty Weigh In on New Stem Cell Strategy." UCSF Today. 25 August 2006. 4 January 2007. <http://pub.ucsf.edu/today/cache/feature/200608247>.

"UCSF Human Embryonic Stem Cell Research Center." University of California, San Francisco. 4 January 2007. <http://escells.ucsf.edu/main/home.asp>.

"United States is Not a Christian Nation." Embassy of Heaven. 6 March 2007. <http://secular.embassyofheaven.com/usa/tripoli.htm>.

"US Governs by 'Coercion,' Iran leader Writes In Open Letter to Americans, Ahmadinejad Urges Pullout from Iraq." MSNBC News Services. Nov 29, 2006. <http://www.msnbc.msn.com/id/15947213/>.

"Want Stem Cells? Head to Singapore." CNet News.com. 21 August 2006. Accessed 28 December <2006.http://news.com.com/2061-11128_3-6107716.html>.

"Welcome to China Stem Cell News." 13 October 2006. Accessed 3 January 2007. <http://www.stemcellschina.com/>.

"What is a Stem Cell?" University of California, Sue and Bill Gross Stem Cell Research Center. 8 January 2007. <http://stemcell.bio.uci.edu/facts/basics.cfm>.

"Wide Range of Possible Treatments Indepth: Genetics and Reproduction Stem cells." CBC News Online. August 24, 2006. Accessed 4 December 2006. <http://www.cbc.ca/news/background/genetics_reproduction/stemcells.html>.

"Windhover's Review of Emerging Medical Ventures." Start up. 1 January 2007. <http://www.windhover.com/contents/monthly/SU0102.HTM>.

BIBLIOGRAPHY B

Aldridge, Susan. "Stem Cell Research Aids Cosmetic and Reconstructive Surgery." American Association for the Advancement of Science 17 February 2005. Accessed 3 January 2006. <http://www.healthandage.com/Home/gm=1!gid1=6899>.

Almeida, Carla. "Brazil Announces US$5 Million for Stem Cell Research." SciDev Net. 5 September 2005. Accessed 3 January 2007. <http://www.scidev.net/News/index.cfm?fuseaction=readNews&itemid=2333&language=1>.

Alterman, Eric. "Neoconning the Media A Very Short History of Neoconservatism." Media Transparency. April 22, 2005. Accessed 4 February 2007. <http://www.mediatransparency.org/story.php?storyID=2>.

Bailey, Ronald. "More Stubborn Facts Are embryos people?" 6 August 2001. <http://www.nationalreview.com/comment/comment-bailey080601.shtml>.

Benac, Nancy. "Poll: Americans Oppose Iraq Troop Surge." Associated Press. 11 January 2007. <http://news.yahoo.com/s/ap/20070111/ap_on_re_us/iraq_ap_poll>.

Berger, Sam. "The Silent Stem Cell Majority." Center for American Progress. February 22, 2006. <http://www.americanprogress.org/issues/2006/02/b1433729.html>.

Bloodworth, Dan. "Re: Collect material from 16 years of Stem Cell Research." Personal interview. 14 November 2006.

Bloodworth, Dan. "Re: Gathering information about Stem Cell Research." Personal interview. 2 August 2006.

Bloodworth, Dan. "Re: Writing a Book about Stem Cell Research." Personal interview. 5 October 2005.

Brown, Nina "The Best Possible Life—Nina Brown's Story." Email. 26 February 2007.

Brown, Rayilyn. "Prentice List and Your Story." Email correspondence. 18 February 2007.

Brown, Rayilyn. Email. "Kicking Some PD Ass in the Heartland." 26 February 2007.

Buchenot, Judy. "Birth of Hope Boy Recovers from Cerebral Palsy after Having Stem Cell Treatment." Liberty Suburban Chicago Newspapers. 31 August 2006. 5 January 2007. <http://chicagosuburbannews.com/story.php?pub=1&sid=61807>.

Bush, George W. "Fact Sheet: Embryonic Stem Cell Research." The White House. 9 August 2001. 1 December 2006. <http://www.whitehouse.gov/news/releases/2001/08/20010809-1.html>.

Bush, George W. "President Bush on Cloning." PBS.org 10 April 2002. 9 August 2006. <http://www.pbs.org/newshour/updates/april02/bush-cloning_4-10.html>.

Bush, George W. "President Discusses Stem Cell Research." The White House. 9 August 2001. 1 December 2006. <http://www.whitehouse.gov/news/releases/2001/08/20010809-2.html>.

Bush, George. "Fact Sheet." United States Department of Human Health and Services. 14 July 2004. 9 August 2006. <http://www.hhs.gov/news/press/2004pres/20040714b.html>.

Campo-Flores, Arian. "Split Remains." Newsweek. Aug 26, 2006. MSNBC.com. 7 November 2006. <http://www.msnbc.msn.com/id/14527419/site/newsweek/>.

Campo-Flores, Arian. "Those Favoring Stem Cell Research Increases to a 73 to 11 Percent Majority." Harris Interactive. September 4 issue of Newsweek. Accessed 9 January 2007. <http://www.harrisinteractive.com/harris_poll/index.asp?PID=488>.

Carter, Jimmy. "Stem Cell News." CAMR. 22 February 2007. <http://www.camradvocacy.org/news_detail.aspx?id=SArch13>.

Chemerinsky, Erwin. "Establishment Clause under Attack." Email to DefCon Members. 6 March 2007.

Cocozzelli, Frank . "An Embryo is Not the Equivalent of a Natural Born Human Being." StemPac.com. May 05, 2006. 4 February 2007. <http://www.stempac.com/weblog/diary/?storyId=566>.

Cocozzelli, Frank. "Catholic Position on Blastocyst Stem Cell Research." Telephone interview. 2 February 2007.

Cocozzelli, Frank. "Facts Checking." Email Correspondence. 6 February 2007.

Cocozzelli, Frank. "Neoconservatism, the Catholic Church and Stem Cells Attack on Science." 15 October 2006. <http://www.talk2action.org/story/2006/10/15/151651/45>.

Cocozzelli, Frank. "Neoconservativism and Opus Dei." Telephone call. 4 February 2007.

Coghlan, Andy. "Blood could generate body repair kit." NewScientist.com News Service. 26 November 2003. Accessed 5 December 2006. <http://www.newscientist.com/article.ns?id=dn4418>.

Conner, Steve. "Hawking Criticises EU States Trying to Ban Stem Cell Research." The Independent Online. 24 July 2006. Accessed 28 February 2006. <http://news.independent.co.uk/world/science_technology/article1193119.ece>.

Cook, Gareth. "U.S. Stem Cell Research Lagging Without Aid, Work Moving Overseas." The Boston Globe. May 23, 2004. Boston.com. 11 December 2006. <http://www.boston.com/news/science/articles/2004/05/23/us_stem_cell_research_lagging?mode=PF>.

Dabu, Christl. "Stem Cell Research and Muslim Law. How A Debate Over Embryos Might Turn Out In Egypt." Christian Science Monitor. June 22, 2005. Accessed 3 January 2006. <http://www.cbsnews.com/stories/2005/06/22/tech/main703569_page2.shtml>.

Davis, Michael. From Tragedy to Triumph. Unpublished manuscript. October 16, 2006.

Defcon America. 28 November 2006. <http://www.defconamerica.
org/about-DefCon/>.

Doerflinger, Richard M. "Science and Ethics: Together Again?" U.S.
Catholic Bishops Life Issues Forum. 26 August 2005. Accessed
8 November 2006. <http://www.usccb.org/prolife/publicat/
lifeissues/082605.htm>.

Dwyer, Sheila. "Dr. Evan Snyder Discusses Advances in A-T
Research." Body1.com. August 18, 2000. Accessed 11
December 2006. <http://www.body1.com/hero/index.
cfm/1/16/1>.

Einhorn, Bruce and Jennifer Veale and Manjeet Kripalani. "Asia Is Stem
Cell Central, Singapore and others are racing to grab the lead
in a promising field." Business Week online. 10 January 2005.
Accessed 27 December 2006. <http://www.businessweek.
com/magazine/content/05_02/b3915052.htm>.

Elder, Robert. "In Houston, a Stem Cell War Room: Scientists and
Activists Gird for a High-Stakes Political Battle." American-
Statesman. 13 June 2005. Accessed 20 February 2007. <www.
statesman.com/metrostate/content/metro/stories/06/
13stemcell.html>.

Elias, Paul. "Stem cells Discovered in Amniotic Fluid." The Associated
Press. 23 August 2006. Accessed 8 January 2007. <http://
news.yahoo.com/s/ap/20070108/ap_on_he_me/stem_cells>.

Faden, Ruth R. and John D. Gearhart. "Facts on Stem Cells." 23
August 2004. Accessed 10 January 2007. <http://www.
washingtonpost.com/wp-dyn/articles/A25071-2004Aug22.
html>.

Fajt, Susan. Personal telephone interview. 15 March, 2007.

Fallon, James, Dr. Email correspondence. "TGFa and Your Book." 24
January 2007.

Finkle, Jim. "Stem Cell Firm Optimistic on Ethical Concerns."
28 August, 2006. <http://maconareaonline.com/news.
asp?id=14971>.

Ford, Gerald. "Stem Cell News." CAMR. 25 April 2002. <http://www.camradvocacy.org/news_detail.aspx?id=SArch14>.

Fox, Maggie. "Human Stem Cells Help Blinded Rats: Study." Washington Post. 21 September 2006. Accessed 12 December 2006. <http://www.advancedcell.com/recent-news-item/human-stem cells-help-blinded-rats-study>.

Goldberg, Maggie. Christopher Reeve Foundation. Email correspondence. 10 January 2007.

Goldman, Steven A. M.D. "Progenitor Cell-Based Myelination of Congenitally Dysmyelinated Brain." University of Rochester Medical Center. 20 August, 2006. <http://www.urmc.rochester.edu/goldmanlab/remyelination.htm>.

Goldman, Steven A. MD. "Perinatal Implantation of Human Glial Progenitor Cells as a Treatment Strategy for the Childhood Myelin Disorders." CSN Foundation. 29 December 2006. <http://www.cnsfoundation.org/site/PageServer?pagename=rch_SGProgRpt>.

Grabmeier, Jeff. "As Stem Cell Debate Heats Up, Public Still Uninformed and Undecided." 12 December 2006. <http://researchnews.osu.edu/archive/stemcell.htm>.

Gross, Cindy-Jo. "Testimony Stem Cell Research." 1 May 2003. Accessed 9 January 2007. <http://www.jewishalliance.org/lte/stem_cell.htm>.

Haverlock, Jim. "My Stem Cell Experiment." 9 January 2007. <http://www.14ushop.com/flyin-blind>.

Haverlock, Jim. "Re: Update to Stem Cell Treatment Story." 9 January 2007.

Heidi Nicholl. "Scientists Discover Cardiac 'Master Cells'." Bionews.org. 27 November 2006. Accessed 13 December 2006. <http://bionews.org.uk/new.lasso?storyid=3272>.

Herman, Linda. "Yvonne's Important Book." Email. 28 February 2007.

Herskovitz, Jon. "S. Korea Stem Cell Pioneer Back in Lab, Inquiry
   Due." The Journal of Turkish Weekly. 12 December 2005.
   Accessed 6 December 2006. <http://www.turkishweekly.net/
   news.php?id=23283>.

Hester, Tom. "Lawmakers Ante $270 Million for Stem Cell Research."
   Star-Ledger Staff. December 15, 2006. Accessed 9 January
   2007. <http://www.nj.com/news/ledger/jersey/index.ssf?/
   base/news-5/1166162511211060.xml&coll=1>.

Holden, Constance. "Stem Cell Alternatives." Science Magazine. 27
   March 2007 <http://www.sciencemag.org>.

Hooker, Richard. "Early Christianity." 23 October 2006. <http://wsu.
   edu/~dee/CHRIST/CHR.HTM>.

Hynes, Dan. "Illinois Poised to Lead on Stem Cell Research."
   Dailysouthtown.com. 28 February, 2007. <http://www.
   dailysouthtown.com>.

Indrajit, Basu. "India Embraces Stem Cell Research."Asia Times
   Online. 5 December 2006.
   <http://www.atimes.com>.

Jagasia, Madan. "Re: Stem Cell Research at Vanderbilt University
   Medical Clinic." Personal interview. 6 September 2006.

Jessica, Pasley. "VUMC Debuts Novel Stem Cell Heart Therapy." The
   Reporter. 16 March 2007. <http://www.mc.vanderbilt.edu/
   reporter/index.html?ID=5408&keywords=heart+stem+cells&
   start=1&end=10>.

Kaarlela, Corinna. "UCSF Receives Funding for Training Grant From
   Stem Cell Institute." 10 April 2006. University of California,
   San Francisco. 4 January 2007. <http://pub.ucsf.edu/
   newsservices/releases/200604108/>.

Kaplan, Karen and Erin Cline. "Stem Cell Limits Have Scientists Seeing
   Double." Alliance for Stem Cell Research. 9 January 2007.
   <http://www.curesforcalifornia.com/page.php?id=316>.

Kessler, John A. "Stem Cells I want to See my Daughter Walk Again." Chicago Tribune. June 2004. Accessed 27 December 2006.

Kessler, John. "Stem Cell Biologist John Kessler Argues for Change in Government Policies." Feinberg School of Medicine. 26 December 2006. <http://www.northwestern.edu/observer/issues/2004-11-04/kessler.html>.

King James Version of the Bible. BibleGateway.com. <http://www.biblegateway.com/>.

Klipstein, Matthew. "TGFa." Email correspondence. 18 January 2007.

Klipstein, Matthew. "Your Book." Email correspondence. 24 January 2007.

Knowlton, Brian. Kissinger Says Victory in Iraq Is Not Possible. The New York Times. Sunday 19 November 2006. Accessed 21 December 2006.

Kounteya Sinha Cloning's out, but Stem Cell R&D will have rules 17 Nov, 2006 IstTimes News Network. 6 December 2006. http://timesofindia.indiatimes.com/articleshow/461473.cms

Kraft, Dina. "Stem Cell Researchers in Israel Warily Eye Debate in Washington." Deep South Jewish Voice. 16 June 2005. Accessed 4 December 2006. <http://deepsouthjewishvoice.blogspot.com/2005/06/israel-file-stem-cell-researchers-in.html>.

Kriegstein, Arnold MD and Prof. Ronald Green. "Stem Cells Created without Destroying Human Embryos." AirTalk, KPCC-FM (NPR), August 24, 2006. Accessed 5 January 2007. <http://pub.ucsf.edu/today/cache/feature/200608247>.

Laitner, Sarah and Clive Cookson. "EU to Fund Embryonic Stem Cell Research." Financial Times. July 24 2006. Accessed 4 December 2006. <http://www.ft.com/cms/s/1d419f90-1b47-11db-b164-0000779e2340.html>.

Lamb, Gregory M. "Stem Cell Research Hinges on States." CBS News.com. 30 November 2006. <http://www.cbsnews.com/stories/2006/02/01/politics/main1269361.shtml>.

Macer, Darryl Ph.D. "Asian Approaches to Stem Cell Research and
    IP Protection." Eubios Ethics Institute." 6 December 2006.
    <http://ipgenethics.group.shef.ac.uk/conference/papers/
    Macer.pdf>.

McAllister, Ted V. "Revolt Against Modernity, Leo Strauss, Eric
    Voegelin, and the Search for a Postliberal Order." University
    Press of Kansas. 4 February 2007. <http://www.kansaspress.
    ku.edu/mcarev.html>.

McCann, Chuck. "My Story about Parkinson's." Personal email.
    October 31, 2006.

McCullagh, Declan. "Congress Plans Scrutiny of Patriot Act." Nwes.
    com. 9 May 2005. Accessed 29 November, 2006. <http://
    news.com.com/Congress+plans+scrutiny+of+Patriot+Act/21
    00-1028_3-5700986.html?tag=nefd.top>.

McGuirk, Rod. "Australia Lifts Ban on Cloning Human Embryos
    for Stem Cell Research." Canadian Press. December 6, 2006.
    CBC News. 27 December 2006. <http://www.cbc.ca/cp/
    health/061130/x113004A.html>.

Mitchell, Steve. "Stem Cells Turned into Organ Precursors." Stem Cell
    Network. 28 October 2005. Accessed 1 January 2007. <http://
    www.stemcellnetwork.ca/news/articles.php?id=869>.

Morrissey, Susan. "States and Stem Cells." Chemical and Engineering
    News. 22 March 2005. 28 December 2006. <http://pubs.acs.
    org/cen/news/83/i12/8312stemcells.html>.

Mummolo, Jonathan. "Scientific Sidestep? Researchers Say That They
    Have Found A Way To Produce Stem-Cell Lines Without
    Destroying Human Embryos." MSNBC.com. 7 November
    2006. http://www.msnbc.msn.com/id/14483409/site/
    newsweek/

Nancy Gibbs, Alice Park, Mike Allen, and Massimo Calabresi,
    "What A Bush Veto Would Mean For Stem Cells," Time.
    24 July 2006. <http://www.whitehouse.gov/news/
    releases/2006/07/20060717-5.html>.

Paine, Thomas. The Age of Reason. New York. Kensington Publishing Corp, 1974.

Peters, Ted Dr. "What is the Embryonic Status of Totipotent and Pluripotent Stem Cells?" 21 December 2006. <http://www.meta-library.net/stemtp/quest2-body.html>.

Philipkoski, Kristen. "Stem-Cell Patient Roasts Lawmaker." Wired News. 3 June 2005. Accessed 20 February 2007. <www.wired.com/news/medtech/0,1286,67728,00.html>.

Porterfield, Andrew. "Stem Cells Stimulated by Natural Growth Factor Reverse Damage, Restore Some Function in Adult Brain." UCI Health.com. 3 January 2007. <http://www.ucihealth.com/News/Releases/StemCells.htm>.

Reagan, Mike and Howard Dean, M.D. "Stem Cell Pro and Con." MSNBC.com. 12 December 2006. <http://cagle.msnbc.com/news/StemCellsProCon/main.asp>.

Reed, Don C. "Chapter by Chapter Book Summary." Telephone interview. 1 February 2007.

Reed, Don C. "Facts Checking and Additional Information." Telephone interview. 18 February 2007.

Reed, Don C. "McNerney in the Morning." Stem Cell Battles. 24 October 2006. <http://www.stemcellbattles.com/Archive%20242_10-24-06%20-%20MCNERNEY%20IN%20THE%20MORNING.htm>.

Reed, Don C. "Shocking Conversation." Email to listserv. 21 March 2007.

Reed, Don C. Email to Listserv. 21 February 2007.

Republican Study Committee. "H.R. 3 — Stem Cell Research Enhancement Act of 2007" Legislative Bulletin. January 10, 2007. 20 February 2007. <http://www.house.gov/hensarling/rsc/lgbullettins07.shtml>.

Ross, Timberly. "Expert Says Cloning Ban Would Hurt Nebraska" Journal Star. 4 March 2007. <http://www.journalstar.com/articles/2007/03/04/news/politics/doc45eb51860179849055 4508.txt>.

Salter, Jim. "Exit Poll Ties Senate Race to Stem Cell Measure." Associated Press. 10 November 2006. <http://news.aol.com/topnews/articles/_a/exit-poll-ties-senate-race-to-stem cell/n20061108164009990010>.

Saltus, Richard. "The Man Who Fixes Brains / Conference Calendar Deadline Friday." The Boston Globe. 27 December 2006. <http://www.pdcaregiver.org/StemCell.html>.

Schneider, Mary. "A Toast to Adult and Cord Blood Stem Cells." Speech given 20 June 2006 in the Senate Russell Office Building 385. 2 January 2007. <http://www.stemcellresearch.org/testimony/20060620_Schneider.htm>.

Schneider, Mary. "Facts Checking." Telephone interview. 23 February 2007.

Schneider, Mary. "Re: Son Infused with Stem Cells by Dr. Joanne Kurtzberg." Telephone interview. 2 January 2007.

Simpson, Taryn. "Living with PD." Personal email. December 1, 2006.

Slack, Gordy. "California Stem Cell Program is Legal: Judge Challengers Vow to Appeal, Making Agency's Future Uncertain." The Scientist. 24 April 2006. 20 February 2007. <http://www.the-scientist.com/news/display/23342/>.

Smith, Peter J. "UK Researcher: Embryonic Stem Cells Have Never Been Used to Treat Anyone and No Plans Exist to do so." Life Site. 4 January 2007. <http://www.lifesite.net/ldn/2006/aug/06082401.html>.

Smith, Shane G. "Outline of my Book." Telephone interview. 2 February 2007.

Smith, Shane G. "Response to Rough Draft." Email. 13 February 2007.

Smith, Shane G. William Neaves and Steven Teitelbaum. "Adult Stem Cell Treatments for Disease?" Science Magazine Vol. 313, p.439, 28 July 2006. 4 February 2007.

Smith, Shane G., William B. Neaves and Steven Teitelbaum. "Research with adult and embryonic cells is essential." 9 January 2007. Op. Ed in St. Louis Dispatch. PDF from author.

Smith, Shane G., William Neaves and Steven Teitelbaum. "Adult Stem Cell Treatments for Disease?" Science Magazine Vol. 313, p.439, 28 July 2006. 4 February 2007.

Snyder, Evan Dr. "Using Stem Cells to Restore Function to Brain Cells Corrupted by Sandhoff Disease." The Children's Neurobiological Solutions. 27 December 2006. <http://www.cnsfoundation.org/site/PageServer?pagename=rch_ESProgRpt06>.

Snyder, Evan. "The New England Journal of Medicine. Interview conducted by Rachel Gotbaum." New England Journal of Medicine. <http://content.nejm.org/cgi/content/full/354/4/321/DC1>.

Snyder, Evan. Telephone Interview. "Re: Confirming Facts about my Research." 4 January 2007.

Snyder, Evan. Telephone Interview. "Re: Writing the Foreword for This Book." October 25, 2006.

Somers, Terri. "How Prop. 71 Came to Life, California Stem Cell Research and Cures Act was Work of Eclectic Group that Included Film Director, Finance Expert, Republican and Researcher." The San Diego Union-Tribune. 19 December 2004. 3 April 2007. <http://www.signonsandiego.com/uniontrib/20041219/news_1n19stemcell.html>.

Somers, Terri. "The City-State Hand-Picks Stem Cell Industry for Economic Growth, and for Scientific Advances." Union-tribune. December 18, 2006. 28 December 2006. <http://www.signonsandiego.com/news/business/biotech/20061218-9999-lz1n18sing.html>.

Stolberg, Sheryl Gay. "Senate's Leader Veers From Bush Over Stem Cells." The New York Times. 29 July 2005. 30 November 2006. <http://www.nytimes.com/2005/07/29/politics/29stem. html?ex=1280289600&en=b97f268f2f13d8d9&ei=5088&part ner=rssnyt&emc=rss>.

Tannenbaum, Jeffrey. "After Dolly Predicts Cloning's Benefits Will Outweigh Perils." Bloomberg.com. 6 September, 2006. <http://www.bloomberg.com/apps/news?pid=20601088&sid =aS2uUvUr1DFQ&refer=muse>.

Tanner, Lindsey. "Heart Valves Grown From Womb Fluid Cells." Associated Press. 15 November 2006. 13 December 2006. <http://www.washingtonpost.com/wp-dyn/content/ article/2006/11/15/AR2006111501033_pf.html>.

Tipton, Sean. "False Claims in GA CAMR.friends Help Needed in Georgia." Email. 1 March 2007.

Tonti-Filippini, Nicholas. "Ignore the Hype in the Cloning Debate." Theage.com.au. September 4, 2006. <http://www.theage. com.au/news/opinion/ignore-the-hype-in-the-cloning-debate/2006/09/03/1157222002193.html>.

Vestal, Christine. "States Eye Stem Cell Research Economics." Stateline. org. 10 January 2006. 30 November 2006. <http://www. stateline.org/live/ViewPage.action?siteNodeId=136&language Id=1&contentId=79291>.

Waters, Rob and John Lauerman. "Scientists Skirt Stem Cell Ban by Building Firewalls" Bloomberg.com June 16, 2006. 5 December 2006. <http://www.bloomberg.com/apps/news?pid=1000008 7&sid=alaONKFjE5N0&refer=top_world_news>.

Weise, Elizabeth. "Dolly was World's Hello to Cloning's Possibilities." USA Today. 4 July 2006. 30 October 2006. <http://www. usatoday.com/tech/science/genetics/2006-07-04-dolly-anniversary_x.htm>.

White, Deborah. "Why Not Give Federal Funds to Churches?" About. com. 1 December 2006 <http://usliberals.about.com/od/ faithinpubliclife/a/Funds_Faith2.htm>.

Williams, Chris. "US Pro-Stem Cell Mission Ready for Fight."
  2 June 2006. The Register. <http://www.theregister.
  com/2006/06/02/congress_stem_cell_delegation/>.

Young, Emma. "MS Damage Repaired by Stem Cells." NewScientist.
  com. 21 January 2003. 9 January 2007. <http://www.
  newscientist.com/article.ns?id=dn3288>.

Zuckman. Jill. "Will Stem Cells be the Key in Races?" Chicago Tribune.
  24 October 2006. 1 March 2007. <http://deseretnews.com/
  dn/view/0,1249,650201249,00.html>.

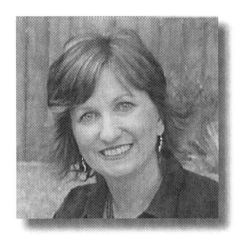

ABOUT THE AUTHOR

Yvonne Perry is a freelance writer, author and keynote speaker who enjoys assisting people on a spiritual path by writing about topics that inspire excellence and uplift the spirit. She is a graduate of American Institute of Holistic Theology where she earned a Bachelor of Science in Metaphysics. Her style of writing is lovingly controversial and challenges people's belief systems in order to help them move past what she calls "Sunday School mentality." She has earned Platinum Expert Author status for her articles on spirituality, death, afterlife, spirit communication, suicide, and politics published on ezinearticles.com.

Everyone has a message they want to share with the world. As a ghostwriter, Yvonne enjoys helping people get their message into a well-written book or article that is ready to publish. She is the owner of Write On! Creative Writing Services—a team of full-time freelance writers located in Nashville, Tennessee. She started the business in 2003 when she left her full-time position as an administrative assistant in the sales and marketing division of a Fortune 500 company. Long gone are the early days of struggling to find writing assignments as a solo writer. By aligning herself and her company with other writers and experts in the field, Perry has networked her company to the top of Google search engines as a premier ghostwriter in Nashville, Tennessee. She and her team stay busy on client projects such as media releases, ghostwriting and editing books, article writing, creating ad copy, and producing business documents. The team provides writing and editing services to individuals and business owners while offering a logical way for large corporations to outsource their writing needs. Thanks to the Internet, the company's reputation has reached international status. If you need a brochure, Web text, business document, career résumé, article or book, visit www.yvonneperry.net.With her wide variety of writing experience that includes impressive résumés, personal and professional bios, high-quality press releases and articles, as well as case studies, proposals and marketing pieces, Yvonne is ready to work with you on your next project.

Under her own name, Perry has authored eleven children's eBooks known as The Sid Series. The books build self-esteem and empower young ones to follow inner guidance and overcome fear. Inspired by her grandchildren, these stories offer valuable messages that support the whole child—body, soul and spirit—and teach environmental responsibility.

She is also the author of a humorous book entitled *Email Episodes* about a woman experiencing an identity crisis as she faces divorce and approaches mid-life with teenagers who are raising reptiles in the basement. Her books are available on her website at www.yvonneperry.net/books.htm

In April 2005, Yvonne released *More Than Meets the Eye: True Stories about Death, Dying and Afterlife,* a book that address topics that many people are not comfortable talking about such as suicide, the near-death experience, end of life decisions, and euthanasia. The book is designed to help people release their fear of death, learn to communicate with those on the other side and comfort someone who is grieving the loss of a loved one. The book is available at Amazon.com. You may read more about the book on Yvonne's website: www.yvonneperry.net/books.htm

Write On! Creative Writing Services publishes a free monthly ezine called *Writers in the Sky Newsletter.* Each electronic issue accepts contributions from writers, poets, book reviewers, authors, publishers and publicists to fill its pages with information about the craft and business of writing, publishing and marketing books. You may send articles, advertorials and announcements to be included in the newsletter. You may subscribe to the newsletter or read current and archived issues online at http://www.yvonneperry.net/Writers-in-the-Sky-Newsletter.html.

Perry began her journey with Toastmasters in January 2002 and has held several officer roles within the club and at Division level. Yvonne has completed the program requirements for the Advanced Leadership Award. She is the past Area 55 Governor and mentor for Century City Club. As a Distinguished Toastmaster (DTM), she is available to speak about the subject of her books as well as a variety of other topics that inspire excellence and uplift the spirit.

As a public speaker, Yvonne puts her skills to good use through her podcast. An extension of her writing company, *Writers in the Sky Podcast* is a weekly podcast about the craft and business of writing in which Yvonne interviews guest authors, publishers, and book marketing experts. Each Friday a new show is uploaded to iTunes.com and is also available as streaming audio on the company's resource-rich blog of information for writers http://yvonneperry.blogspot.com. A list of shows for the current month and a subscription link to the RSS Feed is available on the company's Website: http://www.yvonneperry.net/WritersintheSkyPodcast.htm.

In addition to these ongoing shows and classes, Yvonne has presented at the following places:

- 2005 Galactic Gateway New Age Fair and Wholistic Expo workshop speaker
- Brentwood United Methodist Church - April 2005
- Calling All Authors on Global Talk Radio. Topic: How I started Write On! Creative Writing Services. Tuesday, September 26 2006.
- Century City Club – March 2, 2006
- Elemental Journey with Nic Daniel. Topic: More Than Meets the Eye: True Stories about Death, Dying, and Afterlife. Monday, October 9, @ 7 p.m.
- First Class Flyers Club - November 16, 2005
- FOI (Friends of Nashville) – a near-death experience study group meeting associated with The International Association for Near-Death Studies (IANDS).

- Nashville Newcomer's Club - February 24, 2006
- Podcast Interview with Suzanne Lieurance on her show Freelance Writing: How to Jumpstart Your Career sponsored by the University of Masters – August 8, 2006
- Radio Interview with May Leilana Schmidt on The Universal Spiritual Connection - May 23, 2006
- Radio Interview with Rev. Juliet Nightingale on her show Toward the Light broadcast on BBSRadio.com - March 20, 2006
- University of Masters teleclass August 31, 2006
- Windows to Wellness talk radio (98.9 WRFN-LPFM). Radio Interview with Linda Woods April 9, 2006

On Yvonne's Website http://yvonneperry.net, you will find testimonials, a client list, a link to her blog, writing tele-classes, newsletter and podcast and bios of each of the writers on her team. Her résumé, references, writing samples and books are also available.

Blog: http://yvonneperry.blogspot.com
Web: www.right2recover.net

ANOTHER TITLE BY YVONNE PERRY

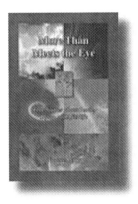

More Than Meets the Eye: True Stories about Death, Dying and Afterlife by Yvonne Perry

Including a commentary by Dr. Aaron Milstone of Vanderbilt University Medical Center, More Than Meets the Eye: True Stories About Death, Dying and Afterlife covers many aspects of the dying and grieving process. Perry uses true stories to look squarely in the face of euthanasia, suicide, near-death experience, post-mortem processes, hospice care, assisting the passing of a loved one, spirit visits from deceased loved ones and other topics people are somewhat reluctant to talk about. The book offers non-religious information and insight to assist people in finding peace about the mysterious process of transitioning back to God/Source. A legal document that may be used as a living will is included in the appendix.

Read more at www.yvonneperry.net/books.htm or purchase at www.amazon.com.

LaVergne, TN USA
02 October 2009
159743LV00001B/149/A